Arrhythmia Interpretation:
ACLS Preparation and Clinical Approach

Ken Grauer, MD, F.A.A.F.P.

Professor, Department of Community Health and Family Medicine
Assistant Director, Family Practice Residency Program
College of Medicine, University of Florida, Gainesville
ACLS Affiliate Faculty for Florida

Dr. Grauer can be reached by:

Mail- Dr. Ken Grauer
　　　Family Practice Residency Progra
　　　625 S.W. 4th Avenue
　　　P.O. Box 147001
　　　Gainesville, Florida 32614

Fax- (352) 332-9154
e-Mail- grauer@fpmg.health.ufl.edu
Web site- http://www.med.ufl.edu/chfm/people/grauer

Daniel Cavallaro, REMT-P

Senior Medical Officer for Lifeguard Air Ambulance
President of the Center for Medical Research, Tampa Florida
Past ACLS National Affiliate Faculty

Dan Cavallaro can be reached by:

e-Mail- danlcav@aol.com

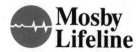

Mosby
Lifeline

St. Louis Baltimore Boston Carlsbad Chicago New York Philadelphia Portland
London Madrid Mexico City Singapore Sydney Tokyo Toronto Wiesbaden

High Point University
Smith Library
833 Montlieu Ave.
High Point, NC 27262-3598

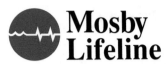

Mosby Lifeline

Dedicated to Publishing Excellence

Vice-President and Publisher: David Dusthimer
Editor-in-Chief: Rick Weimer
Manager, Business Development: Cathy Austin
Senior Assistant Editor: Kay Beard
Project Manager: Doug Bruce
Senior Production Editor: Nadine Fitzwilliam
Book Design: E.L. Graphics
Cover Design: Nancy McDonald

Copyright© 1997 by Mosby-Year Book, Inc.
A Mosby Lifeline imprint of Mosby-Year Book, Inc.

All rights reserved. No part of this publication may be reproduced, stored in a
retrieval system, or transmitted, in any form by any means, electronic, mechanical,
recording, or otherwise, without prior written consent from the publisher.

Permission to photocopy or reproduce solely for internal or personal use is
permitted for libraries or other users registered with the Copyright Clearance
Center, 27 Congress Street, Salem, MA 01970. This consent does not extend to
other kinds of copying, such as copying for general distribution, for advertising or
promotional purposes, for creating new collected works, or for resale.

Printed in the United States of America
Composition by: E.L. Graphics
Printing/binding by: Colour Grafix Group, Inc.

Mosby-Year Book, Inc.
11830 Westline Industrial Drive
St. Louis, Missouri 63146

International Standard Book Number 0-8151-3624-2

96 97 98 99 00 / 9 8 7 6 5 4 3 2 1

In loving memory of my parents,

Samuel and Henrietta Grauer

without whom this book would not have been possible.

Acknowledgments

I am indebted to the following people whose contributions were instrumental to the preparation of this book:

Dan Cavallaro- for his continuing feedback, support, and friendship as I worked through conceptualizing this challenging project.

Kay Beard- for her role as the *major force* (!) in moving this project forth from the drawing board stage to production. Her unwavering support, diligence, and enthusiasm are the reasons this book is reality.

Claire Merrick- for her support and encouragement from above that helped make this project possible. Thank you Claire!

Anita Wofford-Grauer- for being there for me and supporting my efforts during the writing (and seemingly *endless* rewriting) of this book.

Rick Griffin, **Stephanie Ivey**, and **Paul Ivey**- for their friendship and support at the best (!) restaurant in Gainesville- ***Ivey's Grill***- which provided me with the peaceful, pleasant, and inspiring environment for writing (and forever rewriting), and reviewing much of this text (and for the tofu and fruit to keep my coronaries clean). Thanks also to my favorite waiters and waitresses at Ivey's, who truly make up the *best* and friendliest staff anywhere!

Maria Alvarez and **Ray Parris**- those best teachers (and great friends) at the ***Maria Alvarez Imperial Dance Studio***, who have forever been instrumental in helping me to maintain my sanity (and still have fun by dancing) for much of the time I was working on this book.

Judy Niverson- for her friendship and individual attention and support that helped to further improve our dancing (and maintain my sanity).

Barney Marriott, MD, and **William P. Nelson**, MD- *for teaching me more about ECGs than I can ever say.*
The Cardiology staff at Alachua General Hospital (Burt Silverstein, MD; Steve Roark, MD; James O' Meara, MD; and Mike Dillon, MD)- for their tremendous support of me, and for teaching cardiology to our residents.

To *all* of the other excellent cardiologists who have inspired me, and from whom I have learned.

To *all* those who have knowingly (and unknowingly) provided me with tracings and other nuggets of information through the years.
And last but far from least- to *all* the nurses, medical students, residents, and other paramedical personnel who through the years have allowed me to learn by teaching them.

Ken Grauer, MD

About the Authors

KEN GRAUER, M.D., F.A.A.F.P., is a professor in the Department of Community Health and Family Medicine, College of Medicine, University of Florida, and assistant director of the Family Practice Residency Program in Gainesville. He is board certified in family practice, and is ACLS Affiliate Faculty for Florida (and former National ACLS Affiliate Faculty). He is also a former contributor to the American Heart Association ACLS Textbook who served on the Task Force for ACLS Post-Testing. In addition to this book, Dr. Grauer is the principal or sole author of the following books and teaching resources: *ACLS: Rapid Study Card Review* (Third edition, Mosby Lifeline, 1997), *ACLS Rapid Reference* (Third edition, Mosby Lifeline, 1997), *A Practical Guide to ECG Interpretation* (Mosby-Year Book, 1992), *ECG Interpretation Pocket Reference* (Mosby-Year Book, 1992), *Clinical Electrocardiography: A Primary Care Approach* (Second edition- Blackwell Scientific Publications, 1992), and *ACLS Teaching Kit: An Instructor's Resource* (Mosby-Year Book, 1990). His ACLS materials are featured on the Mosby Lifeline CD-ROM products, *ACLS Infobase: The ACLS Omnibus Resource*, and *ACLS Review* (User's Manual and Instructor's Version). He has lectured widely and is primary author of numerous articles on cardiology for family physicians, including several "ECG of the Month" columns that have been published for more than a decade in various primary care journals. He also has served on the Editorial Board of the following journals: Family Practice Recertification, Procedural Skills and Office Technology, and Internal Medicine Alert, Emergency Medicine Alert, and ACLS Alert.

    Dr. Grauer has become well known throughout Florida and nationally for teaching ACLS courses and ECG/arrhythmia workshops to diverse medical audiences including nurses, paramedics, medical students, physicians in training, and physicians in practice. His trademark has always been the ability to simplify otherwise complicated topics into a concise, practical, and easy-to-remember format.

DAN CAVALLARO, REMT-P, is senior medical officer for Lifeguard Air Ambulance, and President of the Center for Medical Research in Tampa, Florida. He is a former ACLS National Affiliate Faculty member, and a former contributor to the American Heart Association ACLS Textbook who served on the Task Force for ACLS Post-Testing. In addition to coauthoring this book, he has coauthored the following teaching resources: *ACLS: Rapid Study Card Review* (Third edition, Mosby Lifeline), *ACLS Rapid Reference* (Third edition, Mosby Lifeline), *ACLS Teaching Kit: An Instructor's Resource* (Mosby-Year Book, 1990), and the Mosby Lifeline ACLS CD-ROM products. Clinically, he has worked in the critical care, emergency medical, and surgical fields for the past 20 years. During that time, he has also been extremely active developing and participating in courses on pre-hospital care and emergency medicine, and has taught in well over 200 ACLS courses.

Contents

Part I- *Basic Arrhythmia Interpretation*

Section 1B- *Systematic Approach*

Section 1C- *SUPRAventricular Rhythms*

Section 1D- *Premature Beats/VT*

Section 1E- *Late Beats/Escape Rhythms*

Section 1F- *Rhythms of Cardiac Arrest*

Section 1G- *AV Blocks- Basic Concepts*

Part II- *Arrhythmia Interpretation:*
Beyond the Core

Section 2A- *Selected Advanced Concepts*

Section 2B- *Aberrant Conduction*

<u>Section 2C</u>- *Pediatric Rhythms*

PREFACE to Arrhythmia Interpretation: ACLS Preparation and Clinical Approach

In order to effectively manage cardiac arrest and emergency cardiac care situations, one must be able to rapidly and accurately diagnose cardiac arrhythmias. The goal of this book is to present a readily mastered approach to aid in rapid recognition and interpretation of the most commonly encountered cardiac arrhythmias.

Much of the material that appears in this book was taken from our previous ACLS publications. This work takes that material an important step further- consolidating and integrating it into a single volume discussion of those arrhythmias that are most likely to be seen by the ACLS provider- as well as by other providers of cardiac care.

How To Use This Book

This book consists of two basic parts, each of which is comprised of a number of sections. Sections may stand alone on their own as concise independent discussion of a key subject area- or they may be read in succession as part of the *sequential* presentation of this book. Key points of interest that are covered in each section are listed below.

Part I of the book is entitled, *"Basic Arrhythmia Interpretation"*. In it we review the basic approach to cardiac arrhythmias. More than 100 illustrative tracings rapidly advance the reader from the fundamentals of rhythm interpretation to a fairly high level of sophistication. Clinical relevance and a problem-solving approach aimed to stimulate and actively recruit reader participation is stressed throughout. Numerous practice tracings (with explained answers) have been included to reinforce concepts discussed- with key points of interest highlighted for readers of *all* levels of expertise and experience. Specific components that comprise Part I include:

- **Section 1A**- *Introductory Concepts/Rate Determination* (in which the essential core concepts that are needed for interpretation are rapidly reviewed).

- **Section 1B**- *Systematic Approach* (in which we present a practical 4-step approach to arrhythmia interpretation- and then illustrate its clinical application).

- **Section 1C**- *SUPRAventricular Rhythms* (in which we present the key features for recognizing the basic supraventricular rhythms- including sinus mechanism rhythms, atrial fibrillation and flutter, PSVT, and junctional rhythms). Review of how vagal maneuvers are used in the diagnostic process completes the discussion in this section.

- **Section 1D**- *Premature Beats/VT* (in which we present the key features for recognizing PACs, PJCs, PVCs, and the various types of ventricular rhythms). Clinical relevance is stressed by discussion and illustration of the differential diagnosis of problematic *WCTs* (wide-complex tachycardias).

- **Section 1E**- *Late Beats/Escape Rhythms* (including discussion of the various types and clinical significance of escape beats and rhythms).

- **Section 1F**- *Rhythms of Cardiac Arrest* (including illustration of ventricular fibrillation, ventricular tachycardia, asystole, PEA, slow idioventricular rhythm, agonal rhythm, and artifact).

- **Section 1G**- *AV Blocks- Basic Concepts* (including discussion of 1°, 2°, and 3° AV block, high-grade block, AV dissociation- and the various mimics of AV block). Clinical implications are stressed throughout.

Part II of this book is entitled, *"Arrhythmia Interpretation: Beyond the Core"*. As suggested by its title, our goal in this second part is to take the reader *beyond* the basics to explore more advanced concepts in arrhythmia recognition. Illustrative clinical examples continually challenge the reader and serve to explain the important points made. Specific components included in Part II are the following:

- **Section 2A**- *Selected Advanced Concepts* (including discussion of the rhythms of digitalis toxicity, ECG manifestations of sick sinus syndrome, rapid atrial fibrillation with WPW, and torsade de pointes).

- **Section 2B**- *Aberrant Conduction* (in which we thoroughly explore the diagnostic criteria for recognizing aberrant conduction and distinguishing it from ventricular ectopy). Application of clinical criteria is illustrated in the assessment of several problematic tachycardias.

- **Section 2C**- *Pediatric Rhythms* (in which we briefly discuss key differences between pediatric arrhythmias and arrhythmias in adults).

Regardless of the reader's clinical background and training, there should be ample material in this book to improve one's ability in arrhythmia interpretation. The basic arrhythmias encountered in ACLS and emergency cardiac care are thoroughly discussed.

For the Reader Who Wants More . . . .

We have recently revised all of our ACLS materials. Now in its fourth edition, our book- *"ACLS: Rapid Review and Case Scenarios"* reviews the American Heart Association ACLS algorithms and their treatment approach in a user-friendly and clinically relevant format according to the new design of the ACLS course.

Similar review of ACLS material according to the new course format is provided in the third edition of our completely revised, *"ACLS: Rapid Study Card Review"*. Simulated code scenarios with detailed explained answers provide optimal preparation for successfully completing the ACLS course (and for managing cardiac arrest).

Finally- concise review of the most important aspects of ACLS is consolidated in our, *"ACLS Rapid Reference"*- the third edition of our reader-friendly pocket reference designed for use at the bedside (and/or last minute preparation for the ACLS course).

Part I

Basic Arrhythmia Interpretation

Section 1A- Introductory Concepts/Rate Determination

Components of Clinical Arrhythmia Interpretation

Conceptually- 3 principal components enter into the process of the *clinical* interpretation of a cardiac arrhythmia:

1) The **ECG Rhythm** itself

2) The **Patient** whose rhythm is being recorded

3) The **Clinician** who is faced with interpreting the tracing and caring for the patient

---

KEY → In approaching the challenge of *clinical* arrhythmia interpretation, we feel it essential to remember what an ECG is- *and what it is not.* An ECG is merely "the graphic representation of the heart's electrical activity"- *nothing more, and nothing less.* Practical application of the information provided from analysis of *any* ECG rhythm strip will depend as much on the other two components of interpretation (i.e., on the patient/clinical situation *and* the interpreter)- as it will on the ECG rhythm itself.

Components of Arrhythmia Interpretation

1) The **ECG Rhythm** itself:
- Hard copy printout of the rhythm in question (that is hopefully of sufficient *duration* to allow proper analysis).
- A view of the rhythm from *additional* monitoring leads.
- Additional tracings on the patient for comparison.
- Selected **12-lead ECGs** on the patient- ideally obtained *prior to-* and *during* the arrhythmia- as well as *after* the arrhythmia has resolved (if treatment is successful).

2) The **Patient** whose rhythm is being recorded:
- Information on **patient specifics**- including age, sex, pertinent medical history, and a list of cardioactive medications that the patient is taking.
- Appreciation of the **clinical setting** in which the rhythm occurs (*See page 7*).

3) The **Clinician/Interpreter** who is caring for the patient:
- The ability to assess information from ECG findings- *in light of* patient specifics/the clinical setting.
- The ability to apply this information in formulating a practical clinical approach to management of the patient.

Note → It will often be difficult to arrive at an optimal clinical interpretation for a given arrhythmia when all you are provided with is a *single* short rhythm strip- especially in the absence of additional clinical information. Unfortunately (and realistically)- you will often *not* have access to as much information as you might like. The point to emphasize is that the more information you are *able* to gather (as suggested above)- the more *accurate* (and *relevant*) your clinical interpretation is likely to be (*See page 9*).

The Clinical Setting :

Importance in Arrhythmia Interpretation (and Management)

Consider the following clinical questions:

1) Is sinus rhythm in excess of 100 beats/minute corrrectly termed sinus *tachycardia* ?

2) Is sinus bradycardia at a rate of 35 beats/minute a *worrisome* finding?

3) Does a patient who presents with atrial fibrillation and a *slow* ventricular response have sick sinus syndrome?

4) Is an alert, *asymptomatic* patient in a sustained WCT *(Wide-Complex Tachycardia)* likely to be in ventricular tachycardia (VT) ?

Hint → The answer to *each* of these four clinical questions can be summarized by the *SAME two words* !

Importance of the Clinical Setting:

Cardiac arrhythmias should *never* be interpreted in a "vacuum" (i.e., in the *absence* of information on patient specifics and the clinical setting). This point is emphasized by our answer to the questions that appear on the front of this card. The *SAME two words* (i.e.,**"depending on"**)- can be used to answer *each* question.

- **Question #1-** The definition of sinus tachycardia may vary- **depending on** the age of the patient. Whereas a sinus rate of ≥100 beats/minute is described as sinus tachycardia in an adult- a *faster* rate (i.e., of 120 beats/minute)- would be perfectly normal for a crying infant (*See pages 357-358*).

- **Question #2-** The clinical significance of bradycardia will vary- **depending on** the setting in which it occurs. Sinus bradycardia at a rate of 35 beats/minute is clearly worrisome when it occurs in an older adult with cardiac symptoms of syncope or heart failure. In this situation, the rhythm suggests *sick sinus syndrome* and the need for a pacemaker. On the other hand, sinus bradycardia at a heart rate of 35 beats/minute is *normal* for an otherwise healthy long distance runner- for whom the slow rate is much more suggestive of superb conditioning (*See pages 93-94*).

- **Question #3-** A slow ventricular response to atrial fibrillation may be an *iatrogenic* finding (i.e., from excessive use of rate-slowing drugs such as digitalis, ß-blockers, verapamil, and/or diltiazem)- **depending on** whether the patient is *receiving* such medication. If not- the occurrence of this rhythm would be *highly suggestive* of sick sinus syndrome (*See page 297*).

- **Question #4-** *Regardless* of the patient's hemodynamic status during the tachycardia- VT is a far more likely cause of a sustained WCT than supraventricular tachycardia (SVT) with either aberrant conduction or preexisting bundle branch block. **Depending on** the history- VT becomes *especially* likely when the patient is an older adult with known underlying heart disease (*See page 181*).

"<u>Tools</u>" *of the Trade*

- *The Systematic Approach*
  - *Calipers*
    - *Additional ECG monitoring leads*
    - *12-lead tracings*
      - *Vagal maneuvers*

<u>**Note**</u> → Discussion on the use of ***Adenosine*** as a diagnostic/therapeutic maneuver in the clinical approach to sustained tachyarrhythmias is deferred until page 135.

"Tools" of the Trade:

The process of *clinical* arrhythmia interpretation is readily accomplished by the use of one or more of the following *"Tools" of the Trade* :

- **The Systematic Approach**- which is probably the *most important* of the tools. We suggest *systematic* assessment of *each* (and *every*) ECG rhythm encountered by the **4 Question Approach** (*See pages 61-86*)- looking for regularity of the rhythm, the presence of P waves, QRS width, and the relationship of P waves to the QRS complex. *Routine use of a systematic approach will prevent omission of any important findings.*

- **Calipers**- which are all too often overlooked as an important tool. *Do NOT be intimidated by the thought of using calipers.* With minimum practice, using calipers quickly becomes a *routine* part of your approach. Rewarding benefits are *immediately* apparent- as rates and regularity are much more easily (and *rapidly* !) determined- and seemingly subtle relationships between atrial and ventricular activity become ever so obvious.

- **Additional ECG monitoring leads/12-lead tracings**- may be helpful in revealing the presence/nature of atrial activity, clues to QRS morphology, and/or additional viewpoints for assessing QRS interval duration (since the QRS may appear deceptively narrow in certain leads- but not in others). It is important to emphasize that assessment of a given arrhythmia may be exceedingly difficult if one is only provided with a rhythm strip obtained from a *single* monitoring lead.

- **Vagal maneuvers (*i.e., carotid massage, Valsalva*)**- may help diagnostically and/or therapeutically- either by *converting* PSVT- and/or by *slowing* the ventricular response of other supraventricular arrhythmias enough to allow detection/recognition of atrial activity that had previously been concealed (*See pages 135-138*).

ECG <u>*Fundamentals*</u>

Before launching into clinical description of specific cardiac arrhythmias and our clinical approach to interpretation- a number of fundamental terms and concepts should be clarified. We do this on the pages that follow in this section. Topics covered include:

- The Pathway of Normal Conduction (*Page 13*)
- The Speed of Conduction (*Page 15*)
- ECG Waveforms (*Page 17*)
- ECG Intervals (*Page 19*)
- The QRS Complex (*Page 21*)
- Mechanical and Electrical Activity (*Page 23*)
- ECG Monitoring- *Static* vs *Dynamic* Recording (*Page 25*)
- ECG Monitoring Leads- *Leads Most Commonly Preferred* (*Page 27*)
- QRS Nomenclature (*Pages 29-36*)
- Technical Aspects- ECG Grid Paper (*Page 37*)
- Calculation of Rate (*Pages 39-46*)
- The **'Rule of 300'**- Calculation of Rate (*Page 47*)
- Rate calculation- *When the R-R interval is NOT an exact number of boxes* (*Page 49*)
- Rate calculation- *When the R-R interval is IRREGULAR* (*Page 51*)
- Rate calculation- *When the rhythm is regular and SLOW* (*Page 53*)
- Rate calculation- *When the rhythm is regular and FAST* (*Page 55*)
- The *'**Every OTHER Beat' Method** (*Page 57*)
- ECG Terminology- Use of <u>*Arrhythmia*</u> or *Dysrhythmia*? (*Page 59*)

ECG Fundamentals

Although the fundamentals reviewed in this section
do need to be stated-
we realize that many of these concepts
are already well known
to many of our readers.

If this is the case, feel free to *rapidly* pass through
the pages in this section-

*- but PLEASE do NOT skip them entirely
(as more advanced "Pearls" are sprinkled throughout!).*

Beginning with **Section 1B** (on page 61)
we present and develop
our ***Systematic Approach to Arrhythmia Interpretation***-
and then immediately launch into the ***Basic Rhythms***.

The Pathway
of <u>Normal Conduction</u>

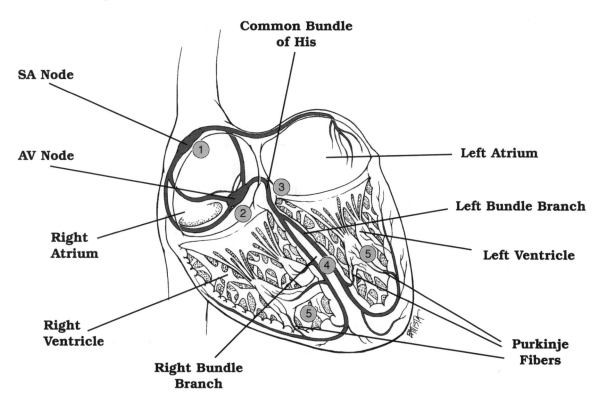

<u>**Question**</u> → In which atrium does the pathway of normal conduction begin? (<u>HINT</u>- *In which atrium is the SA node?*).

The Pathway of Normal Conduction

ECG complexes are a reflection of the heart's *electrical* activity. The electrical activity originates in the **SinoAtrial (SA) node**- the principle pacemaker of the heart. Anatomically- the SA node is located in the upper portion of the *right* atrium (**1**)- *which is why the RIGHT atrium will normally depolarize BEFORE the left atrium.*

In otherwise healthy adults, the SA node will normally discharge at a rate of between 60 to 100 beats/minute- which defines the limits of **normal sinus rhythm (NSR)**. With each electrical discharge, the wave of electrical activity begins on its path through the specialized cells of the heart's conduction system:

- Following discharge of the SA node, the electrical impulse is carried by specialized conduction fibers to the *left* atrium- and *through* the right atrium to the **AtrioVentricular (AV) node**- at which point the electrical impluse is *momentarily* delayed (**2**).

- Following momentary delay in the AV node- the electrical impulse now enters the *ventricular* conduction system- which begins as the **bundle of His** (**3**)- and then divides into **right** and **left bundle branches** (**4**).

- From the bundle branches, electrical activity is carried to ventricular muscle itself *throughout* the heart over the intricate network of specialized **Purkinje fibers** (**5**)- leading to *near* simultaneous activation of the right and left ventricles.

> **Note** → Mechanical contraction of the heart follows electrical activation.

The <u>Speed</u> of Conduction

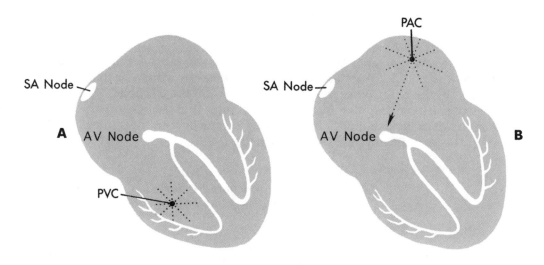

PVC-Premature **V**entricular **C**ontraction
PAC-Premature **A**trial **C**ontraction

<u>**Question**</u> → Why do PVCs produce *wide* ECG complexes ?
(i.e., *Why should it take longer than usual for a PVC
to depolarize the ventricles?*).

The Speed of Conduction

It should be emphasized that the speed at which the electrical impluse travels through specialized cells of the heart's conduction system is *much* more rapid (up to 100 times faster)- than travel over nonspecialized atrial or ventricular tissue. This is the reason why electrical depolarization of the heart is normally accomplished so rapidly and efficiently- and why the QRS of a normal ECG complex is *narrow*.

A number of conditions may alter this process. Among the most common ECG abnormalities are **premature** (i.e., *early* occurring) **ectopic impulses-** in which electrical activity originates from a location in the heart *other than* (i.e., *ectopic* from) the SA node. Three possibilities exist. The premature ectopic impulse may originate from 1) elsewhere in the atria; 2) from somewhere *within* the AV node itself; or 3) from a focus somewhere in the ventricles. Depending on its site of origin this ectopic impluse will be termed:

- a **PAC** (**P**remature **A**trial **C**ontraction)
- a **PJC** (**P**remature **J**unctional **C**ontraction)
- a **PVC** (**P**remature **V**entricular **C**ontraction)

Note → The reason that **PVCs** produce a *widened* ECG complex (that looks much different than normally conducted beats)- is that the ectopic focus originates *outside* of the heart's specialized conduction system (See *Figure A on page 15*). As a result, the electrical impulse begins on its path of conduction from an area of *nonspecialized* ventricular tissue. It therefore takes a much different path- and requires much longer to depolarize the myocardium.

In contrast, **PACs** typically produce a *narrow* ECG complex that is usually quite similar in appearance to normally conducted beats. This is because PACs most often are conducted in a similar manner as normal beats (*Figure B on page 15*). Once the atrial impulse arrives at the AV node- it can now be conducted down the normal pathway. (**PJCs** originate from *within* the AV node- so that they also usually produce a narrow, normal-appearing ECG complex.)

ECG <u>Waveforms</u>

Components of the ECG Complex:

- The **P wave**
    - The **QRS complex**
        - The **T wave** (and **U wave**)

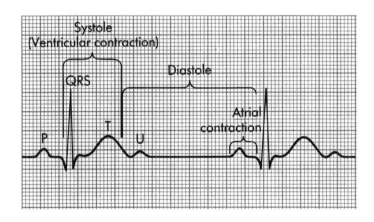

Question → Does the ECG rhythm recorded on a monitor reflect *mechanical* or *electrical* activity?

ECG Waveforms

A normal ECG complex is made up of 3 principal waveforms: the P wave, QRS complex, and T wave. These waveforms reflect the occurrence of *electrical* events in the cardiac cycle. Specifically:

- The **P wave**- reflects *atrial* depolarization

   - The **QRS complex**- reflects *ventricular* depolarization

      - The **T wave**- reflects ventricular *repolarization*

Occasionally a **U wave** may also be seen as a small, usually positive deflection that follows the T wave- and is thought to represent the terminal phase of ventricular repolarization (*See Figure on page 17*).

KEY → Electrical events of the cardiac cycle should *NOT* be confused with their *mechanical* counterparts. Contraction and relaxation of the cardiac chambers are *mechanical* events- that temporally *follow* electrical activation (i.e., depolarization) of these chambers.

For illustrative purposes, we indicate the *approximate* timing of mechanical events in the cardiac cycle on the preceding page. Mechanical **systole** (i.e., ventricular contraction) begins *just after* the onset of the QRS complex- and continues through most of the T wave. **Diastole** (i.e., ventricular relaxation and filling) begins after systole is complete- and culminates with *atrial* contraction (which is seen in the Figure to follow the P wave). Inscription of the next QRS complex marks the approximate onset of the next mechanical systole.

ECG *Intervals*

Three *KEY* intervals are encompassed within the ECG complex. They are:

- The **PR interval**

  - The **QRS complex** (the duration of which is really an interval)

  - The **QT interval**

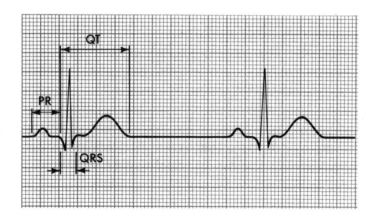

Question → What electrical events occur within the time period encompasssed by the **PR interval** ? *Can you guess where the electrical impulse usually spends the most time during this interval?*

ECG Intervals

- **The PR Interval** → comprises the time from the onset of atrial depolarization (beginning of the P wave)- until the onset of ventricular depolarization (beginning of the QRS complex). Conduction during the first portion of the PR interval is rapid because it occurs over specialized fibers in atrial tissue. Conduction slows down significantly as the electrical impulse passes through the AV node. The physiologic purpose of this relative delay in conduction is to allow the atria adequate time to contract and empty their contents into the ventricles (i.e., to deliver the "atrial kick") prior to the onset of ventricular systole. Clinically, the result is that a major portion of the PR interval is taken up by the time required for the electrical impulse to get through the AV node.

- **The QRS Interval** → is the time that it takes for ventricular depolarization. In healthy subjects who are in sinus rhythm, the QRS complex is usually "narrow"- a result of the *rapidity* with which the electrical impulse is normally transmitted through specialized fibers of the ventricular conduction system. Any condition that prolongs the process of ventricular activation will increase the duration of the QRS interval- *and in so doing may produce QRS widening.*

- **The QT Interval** → is the period from the beginning of ventricular depolarization (onset of the QRS complex)- until the end of ventricular repolarization (end of the T wave). During the initial portion of this interval the heart is *completely refractory* to all premature stimuli (**absolute refractory period**). *Partial* refractoriness of the conduction system is seen during the latter portion of this interval- *the clinical significance of which is discussed on pages 321-322.*

The <u>Q</u>RS Complex

As emphasized on Page 20- the QRS portion of the ECG complex should normally be *narrow*. This is because of the rapid and *efficient* transmission of the electrical impulse over specialized tissues of the ventricular conduction system.

Normal Circumstances
(*Narrow* QRS)

QRS Widening

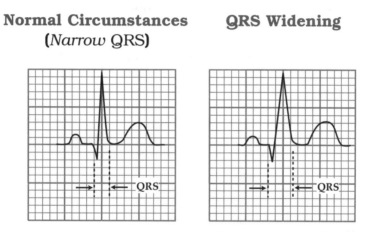

- **<u>Question</u>** → Can you think of a situation in which the QRS complex will be *wide* (i.e., in which ventricular depolarization will take longer)- *despite* transmission of the electrical impulse over the normal AV nodal conduction pathway?

> <u>HINT</u>- Consider the components of the normal conduction pathway (reviewed on pages 13-14)- *and what might go wrong* (i.e., to *delay* transmission of the electrical impulse through the ventricles).

Answers:

As discussed (and illustrated) on page 13, the normal conduction pathway originates in the **SA node**. From there the electrical impulse *sequentially* travels through specialized fibers in atrial tissue- to (and through) the **AV node**- into the **bundle of His**- and then down the **right** and **left bundle branches**- ultimately entering the intricate **Purkinje fiber network** that spreads *throughout* the heart (and makes possible *near* simultaneous activation of the right and left ventricles). Problems with conduction and/or transmission of the electrical impulse may occur *anywhere* along this pathway.

- Difficulty may arise in conduction of the electrical impulse through the atria (or through the AV node)- which might be expected to *slow* conduction (and *delay* arrival) of the electrical impulse to the ventricles. The result will be *lengthening* of the **PR interval**.

- Transmission of the electrical impulse through the AV node may be more severely impaired- so that one or more atrial impulses may *not* get through at all (i.e., there may be **AV "block"**- in which case one or more P waves on the ECG will *not* be followed by a QRS complex).

- Transmission of the electrical impulse through the AV node may occur normally- but conduction may be impaired (or blocked) at a more *distal* site. For example, the right or left **bundle branch** may be **blocked**- in which case the electrical impulse will necessarily travel first down the *unblocked* bundle branch. As a result, ventricular activation will no longer occur in a coordinated and *near* simultaneous manner. Instead, the ventricle innervated by the intact (i.e., *unblocked*) bundle branch will be activated first- with activation of the other ventricle proceding in much *slower* fashion (as electrical activity travels at greatly reduced speed through unspecialized fibers of the "blocked" ventricle). The overall process of ventricular depolarization is therefore *delayed*- and the QRS complex is *widened*. (Note - We discuss criteria for determining QRS widening on pages 79-82).

Mechanical and Electrical Activity

As emphasized on pages 17-18- **mechanical events** in the cardiac cycle (i.e., contraction and relaxation of the cardiac chambers) will normally follow closely after completion of **electrical events** (i.e., after depolarization and repolarization of the atria and ventricles). *Electrical* activity of the heart is represented graphically by the ECG waveforms (i.e., the P wave, QRS complex, and T wave). *Mechanical* activity of the heart is reflected by clinical parameters such as the presence of a pulse, blood pressure, and cardiac output.

- **Question** → Can you think of situations in which *effective* mechanical activity does not occur- *despite* the presence of *electrical* activity (i.e., an ECG complex) on the monitor?

    HINT- Think of the various cardiac rhythms of cardiac arrest.

- **Additional Question** → For which cardiac rhythm will there be *neither* electrical *nor* mechanical activity?

There are several situations in which there is definite evidence of *electrical* activity (i.e., in the form of an ECG rhythm on the monitor)- but no clear evidence of *mechanical* activity (i.e., the patient is *pulseless*). These situations primarily occur in the setting of cardiac arrest. They include:

- **Ventricular fibrillation (V Fib)**

- **Pulseless VT (ventricular tachycardia)**

- **Pulseless Electrical Activity (PEA) rhythms**- a heterogeneous group of rhythms that was previously classified under the term *"EMD"* (i.e., *Electro-Mechanical Dissociation*)

- **Agonal rhythm**- also known as a "dying heart" rhythm

> Clinically- *NONE* of these rhythms are compatible with life- since *none* are associated with any meaningful cardiac output. (*ECG diagnosis of these rhythms of cardiac arrest is discussed on pages 211-234*).

> **Note** → The one cardiac rhythm for which there will be *neither* electrical activity- *nor* mechanical activity- is **asystole** (i.e., a *"flat line"* rhythm in which ECG waveforms are completely absent- *See page 215*).

ECG <u>Monitoring</u>

- *Static* versus *dynamic* recording -

<u>Clinically</u>- *electrical* activity of the heart is displayed in one of two ways: 1) as a **static**- or 2) as a **dynamic** ECG recording. The latter method refers to *ongoing* monitoring of an ECG rhythm (i.e., *dynamic* recording)- a process routinely performed for patients on telemetry. In contrast, *static* recording entails generation of a *hard copy* printout of the rhythm in question (most commonly referred to as a "rhythm strip").

> **<u>Problem</u>** → Imagine you were caring for the patient whose rhythm is shown below.

Lead MCL-1

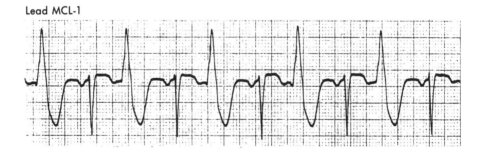

> - What would the *advantage* be of monitoring this patient on telemetry? What is the *drawback* of *exclusively* using this *dynamic* method for ECG monitoring (i.e., without *also* obtaining at least some hard copy ECG recordings)?

ECG Monitoring- **STATIC and DYNAMIC**

The obvious advantage of monitoring a patient on **telemetry** (i.e., *dynamic* monitoring) is the ability to observe *moment-to-moment* changes in the cardiac rhythm. Telemetry monitoring clearly facilitates assessing the need for treatment- since it enables *immediate* correlation of the patient's current cardiac rhythm with the clinical situation. If at *any* time during such monitoring the patient's rhythm (and/or hemodynamic status) changes- appropriate action can be then taken. In addition, the *clinical response* to any treatment measures instituted will be *immediately* seen when the patient is on telemetry- simply because the process of monitoring is continually *ongoing.* In contrast, it is clearly more difficult to assess the need for therapy and the response to intervention when all one is given is a *static* ECG rhythm strip obtained at some earlier time.

> *For example*- it is obvious that every other beat in the rhythm on page 25 is *different* (i.e., wider and oppositely directed compared to the sinus beats- reflecting the fact that every other beat is a PVC). If this particular patient was on telemetry, it would be easy to determine if he/she was symptomatic from the rhythm- simply by history and physical examination. If treatment was indicated- one could then see *right away* if it was effective (depending on whether or not the PVCs went away).

On the other hand, if a patient is monitored *exclusively* by telemetry- there will be a lack of hard copy documentation for events and arrhythmias that occur. Subtleties in ECG interpretation often become apparent *only* after careful analysis of static (i.e., hard copy) recordings- and/or after comparison of a current strip with prior tracings. Maintenance of an updated log of printed *sequential* rhythm strips- in conjunction with *ongoing* telemetry monitoring- are therefore *both* needed for optimal assessment (and documentation) of a patient's clinical course and response to treatment.

ECG *Monitoring Leads*

- *Leads Most Commonly Preferred* -

Return to the rhythm on page 25. The designation- **Lead MCL$_1$** - that appears in the upper left-hand corner of this tracing indicates the **monitoring lead** from which this rhythm strip was recorded. Although details regarding specifics for how to obtain each of the various monitoring leads (i.e., lead placement guidelines, anatomic landmarks, etc.) extends beyond the scope of this text- a number of basic principles should be stated:

- The lead that is chosen for monitoring should always be clearly indicated (as it is in the upper left-hand corner of the rhythm strip shown on page 25).

- Certain monitoring leads are clearly preferable to others- depending on which ECG features are being sought (i.e., the presence and/or nature of P waves, QRS morphology, etc.)

- *"MORE leads are better than one."* The *electrical* viewpoint selected for displaying any given arrhythmia will be *limited* (almost by definition)- if ECG information is *only* provided from a *single* monitoring lead.

- The *monitoring* leads most commonly *preferred* in clinical practice are **leads II - MCL$_1$**- and **MCL$_6$**. Which one (or more) of these leads are selected for monitoring of *any* given patient should depend on specific needs of the clinical situation (*See page 28*).

Preferred Leads for ECG Monitoring:

- **Lead II-** is probably the lead most commonly selected for ECG monitoring. It offers the advantage of providing an excellent look at atrial activity (and **P wave morphology**). Unfortunately, it is of *NO use* for evaluating QRS morphology when P waves are absent and the etiology of a beat or rhythm is uncertain. Thus, lead II is *NOT* at all helpful for distinguishing between ventricular ectopy and aberrant conduction.

- **Lead MCL$_1$-** is an excellent monitoring lead that usually provides helpful information on both the nature of atrial activity and on QRS morphology. The viewpoint of the QRS complex afforded by this *RIGHT-sided* monitoring lead is generally comparable to that of lead V$_1$ on a 12-lead ECG.

- **Lead MCL$_6$-** is an all-too-often *underused* lead in clinical practice. Although usually *not* helpful for identifying the nature of atrial activity- lead MCL$_6$ may provide *invaluable* information for assessment of QRS morphology- especially when the etiology of a rhythm is uncertain from inspection of lead MCL$_1$. The viewpoint of the QRS complex afforded by this *LEFT-sided* monitoring lead is generally comparable to that of lead V$_6$ on a 12-lead ECG.

> **Author's Preference** → We generally prefer to monitor patients *initially* with an **MCL$_1$ lead**- especially when P waves are well seen in this lead and one is *certain* that the rhythm is sinus. Depending on needs of the clinical situation (i.e., the need for a better/different look at *atrial* activity- *and/or* for additional assessment of *QRS* morphology)- we might then switch to *either* a lead **II** or **MCL$_6$** monitoring lead.

*Q*RS <u>*Nomenclature*</u>

The **QRS complex** is subject to great variability in appearance. As an aid to communication, a system has been developed that allows us to *verbally* describe the morphologic appearance of virtually any QRS complex- even to persons who do *not* have the tracing in front of them!

> **Note** → Recognition of relatively small differences in QRS morphology may sometimes be important. For example, consider the four complexes below:

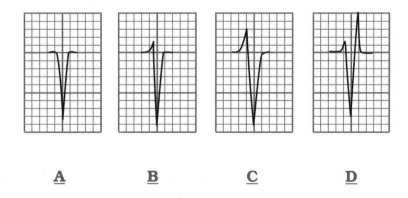

<u>**A**</u>   <u>**B**</u>   <u>**C**</u>   <u>**D**</u>

Do these complexes look the same? How would you *describe* their differences?

Answer

It is obvious that complexes **A**, **B**, **C**, and **D** are all quite different from each other- in relatively small, yet nonetheless *important* ways. Rather than attempting verbal description of the relative height of small or large, upright and negative deflections- *Isn't it easier to simply label each complex with a lettered designation as we have done below each figure?*

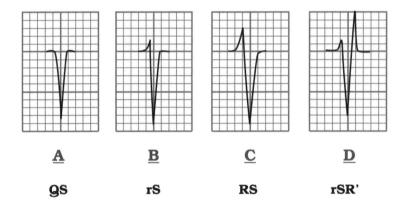

A	**B**	**C**	**D**
QS	**rS**	**RS**	**rSR'**

Suggestion → *Return to this card AFTER reviewing the material presented on pages 31-36.* It should now be apparent how the system for **QRS nomenclature** allows us to specify fine differences noted between each of the above complexes. For example, complexes A and B are both relatively *narrow.* In addition to the presence of a small initial r wave, complex **B** is distinguished from complex **A** by the fact that it has a slightly *deeper* S wave. Complex **C** is clearly *wider* than complex B- and its initial R wave is clearly taller and fatter. Complex **D** is relatively wide- and is distinguished from the still wider complex C and narrower complex B by the addition of an *extra* deflection (i.e., an R').

QRS Nomenclature

(Continued)

The system for QRS nomenclature is comprised of **6 *basic* rules**. The first 3 of these rules are illustrated in the Figure below.

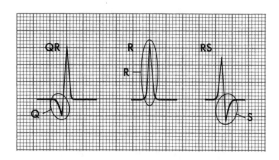

- **Rule #1-** The first *downward* deflection of the QRS complex is termed a **Q** wave.

- **Rule #2-** The first *upward* deflection is termed an **R** wave.

- **Rule #3-** The downward deflection that *follows* the R wave is termed an **S** wave- *IF* it descends *below* the baseline.

Note → It should be apparent from the above Figure that *not* every QRS complex necessarily has all three components (i.e., a Q wave, R wave, and S wave). Thus, the first complex in this Figure is a **QR** complex- the second is an **R** complex- and the third is an **RS** complex.

QRS Nomenclature (Continued):

- **<u>Rule #4</u>-** Large deflections are denoted by capital letters. *Smaller deflections* (i.e., deflections that do *not* exceed 3 mm [= 3 little boxes]) *are denoted by lower-case letters.*

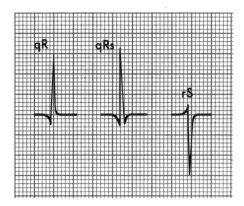

<u>Note</u> → The Figure above depicts **qR**, **qRs**, and **rS** complexes. The initial deflection of each of these complexes is *small* (i.e., *not more* than 3 mm in amplitude)- and followed by a deflection in the *opposite* direction of much greater amplitude. The middle complex is terminated by a small negative deflection.

QRS Nomenclature

(Continued)

- **Rule #5-** If there is a second positive deflection, it is given a *prime* notation: **R'** or **r'** (depending on its size). A third positive deflection is designated an **R"** (or **r"**). Similarly, a second S wave (if present) is termed an **S'** or **s'**.

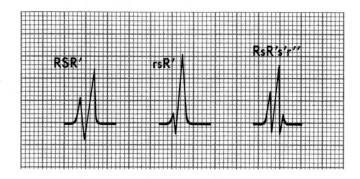

> **Note** → The Figure above depicts QRS complexes with more than one positive or negative deflection.

QRS Nomenclature (Continued):

- **Rule #6-** When there is only a negative deflection, the configuration is called a **QS** complex. This is because of our inability to differentiate between a Q wave, an S wave- or a combination of both when no R wave is present.

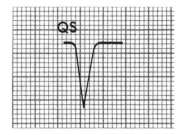

> **Note** → The Figure above depicts a **QS** complex. In the absence of a positive deflection (R wave)- it is impossible to tell if the negative deflection represents a Q wave, an S wave, or some combination of both.

QRS *Nomenclature*

(Continued)

Practice → Use the system for QRS nomenclature to label the following complexes. *Write out your answers.*

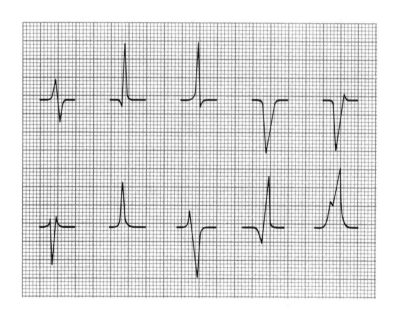

Answers:

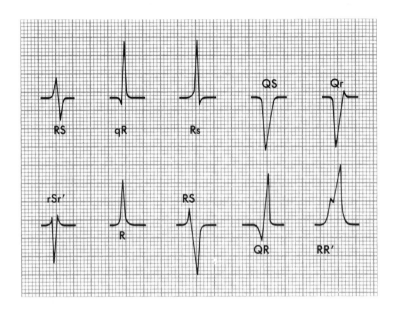

> **Note** → Clinically, determination of the *initial direction* of the QRS complex may be extremely important- since an initial *downward* (negative) deflection on a 12-lead ECG may signify myocardial infarction (as in the qR, QS, Qr and QR complexes above)- whereas a positive deflection will not.
>
> Regarding the last complex in the above Figure, the correct designation is RR' (as shown)- *rather than* RsR' (since the small downward drop that is seen to occur *between* the R and R' waves does *not* descend below the baseline).

Technical Aspects:

- ECG Grid Paper -

With *Introductory Concepts* behind us- we now turn our attention to the process of rhythm determination. The first step in this process is the calculation of rate- which is easily done with the assistance of **ECG grid paper**. Virtually all electrocardiograms and rhythm strips are recorded on this special type of paper- that is usually quite similar to that shown below:

ECG Grid Paper

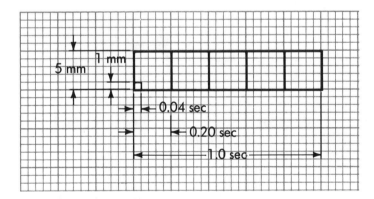

Question → What are the dimensions of each *small* box on ECG grid paper? of each *large* box? How much time does it take for the recording of 5 large boxes?

ECG Grid Paper

As is apparent from the Figure on page 37 -**ECG grid paper** is made up of *large* and *small* boxes. Each *SMALL box* is a square that measures one millimeter (mm) on each side. Each *LARGE box* is a square that is comprised of five little boxes (or 5 mm) on each side.

ECGs are recorded at a standard speed of **25 mm/second**. This means that 25 small boxes (*or 5 large boxes*) of ECG grid paper will be used with each passing second as the tracing is recorded. It follows that the amount of time required to record the contents inscribed on *one* **SMALL box** of ECG grid paper = 1/25th second = **0.04 second**.

From the Figure it can be seen that **time** (in seconds) is displayed along the *longitudinal* axis of ECG grid paper- while **amplitude** (in millimeters) is displayed along the *vertical* axis.

Therefore, the dimensions for *each* **SMALL box** on ECG grid paper are **0.04 second** in time- and **1 millimeter** in amplitude.

From the above- it should follow that the amount of time required to record the contents inscribed on *one **LARGE box*** of ECG grid paper (i.e., *the time equivalent of 5 small boxes*) = **0.20 second** (i.e., *0.04 second X 5 = 0.20 second*).

Therefore, the dimensions for *each* **LARGE box** on ECG grid paper are **0.20 second** in time- and **5 millimeters** in amplitude.

Calculation of <u>Rate</u>

- *Use of ECG Grid Paper* -

Clinically apply the information discussed on pages 37-38 to the example below. Note in this tracing that a QRS complex occurs with each *large* box.

<u>Problem</u> → Calculate the **rate** for the rhythm below. Express your answer in the number of **beats** (i.e., QRS complexes) that occur *per* **minute**.

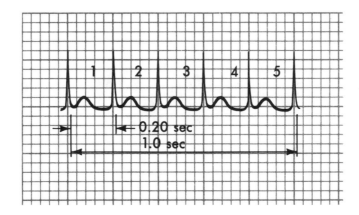

Answer:

As shown in the Figure on page 39- a QRS complex is seen to occur with each *large* box. This means that the **R-R interval** (i.e., the amount of time *between* the recording of each QRS complex) must be 0.20 second. This in turn means that **5 QRS complexes** are being recorded with *each* passing **second** (i.e., 0.20 second X 5 = 1.0 second).

Since there are **60 seconds** in a minute- the heart rate for the example shown on page 39 must therefore be:

5 beats (or complexes) occurring per second
X **60** seconds per minute
—————
= **300 beats/minute**

Calculation of <u>*Rate*</u>

(*Continued*)

As derived (and illustrated) on pages 39-40- if a QRS complex occurred every large box- then the heart rate would be 300 beats/minute.

> <u>*Question*</u> → What would the heart rate be if the rhythm was *regular*- and the R-R interval was ***two*** large boxes?

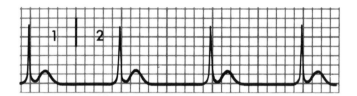

HINT- Since the R-R interval in the above example is *twice* as long as the R-R interval on page 39 (i.e., it is now **2** large boxes or 0.40 second in duration)- *Wouldn't you expect the heart rate to be HALF as fast?*

Answer:

The *thought process* we enlist to determine the rate for this example is suggested by the *HINT* that appears on page 41. It goes as follows:

- We know that the rate of the rhythm on page 39 is **300** beats/minute. We also determined that the R-R interval for that tracing was one *large* box (or 0.20 second) in duration.

   - The R-R interval for the rhythm that appears on page 41 is **twice** as long (i.e., 2 large boxes or 0.40 second in duration).

      - The heart rate for the rhythm that appears on page 41 must therefore be *HALF* as fast as the rate for the rhythm on page 39-

         - or 300 ÷ 2 = **150** beats/minute.

Calculation of <u>Rate</u>

(*Continued*)

<u>*Question*</u> → What would the heart rate be if the rhythm was *regular-* and the R-R interval was ***three*** large boxes?

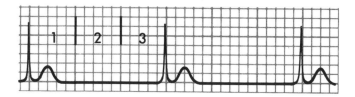

<u>HINT</u>- Since the R-R interval in the above example is *three* times as long as the R-R interval on page 39 (i.e., it is now **3** large boxes or 0.60 second in duration)- *Wouldn't you expect the heart rate to be ONE THIRD as fast?*

Answer:

If instead of a QRS occurring with *each* large box (as shown on page 39) -it took *THREE times* as long (i.e., 3 large boxes- or 0.60 second) to record each QRS complex- then the heart rate should be *one THIRD* as fast. This means that the rate for the rhythm on page 43 should be 300 ÷ 3 = **100** beats/minute.

Calculation of *Rate*

(Continued)

Question → What would the heart rate be if the rhythm was *regular-* and the R-R interval was **five** large boxes?

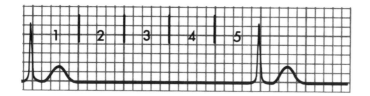

HINT- Since the R-R interval in the above example is *five* times as long as the R-R interval on page 39 (i.e., it is now **5** large boxes or 1.0 second in duration)- *Wouldn't you expect the heart rate to be ONE FIFTH as fast?*

Answer:

If instead of a QRS occurring with *each* large box (as shown on page 39)- it took *FIVE times* as long (i.e., 5 large boxes- or 1.0 second) to record each QRS complex- then the heart rate should be *one FIFTH* as fast. This means that the rate for the rhythm on page 45 should be 300 ÷ 5 = **60** beats/minute.

The "Rule of 300"

- Calculation of Rate -

It should be apparent from the last few examples that heart rate can *rapidly* and *accurately* be determined by the following method:

> - **Dividing 300** *by the number of* **large boxes** *in the* **R-R interval**.

We call this method the **"Rule of 300"**.

> **Note** → The *'Rule of 300'* works best when the rhythm is *regular.*

The "Rule of 300"

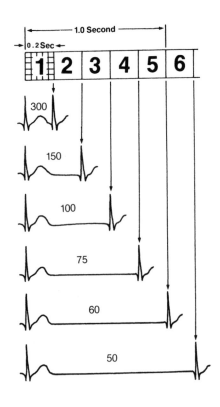

Provided that the rhythm is regular (or at least almost regular)- *heart rate can be estimated by **dividing 300** by the number of **large boxes** in the **R-R interval**.* This rule is schematically illustrated in the accompanying Figure.

Thus- if a QRS complex were to occur *every* **large box**- the heart rate would be **300** beats/minute (*See page 39*). If the R-R interval was *twice* as long (i.e., **2** large boxes)- then the heart rate would be 300 ÷ 2 = **150** beats/minute.

- a QRS every **3** large boxes- . . . a rate of 300 ÷ 3 = **100** beats/minute
- a QRS every **4** large boxes- . . . a rate of 300 ÷ 4 = **75** beats/minute
- a QRS every **5** large boxes- . . . a rate of 300 ÷ 5 = **60** beats/minute
- a QRS every **6** large boxes- . . . a rate of 300 ÷ 6 = **50** beats/minute

Calculation of <u>Rate</u>

- When the R-R interval is NOT an exact number of boxes -

<u>Problem</u>→ Estimate the heart rate for the two examples shown below. Assume in each case that the rhythm was regular.

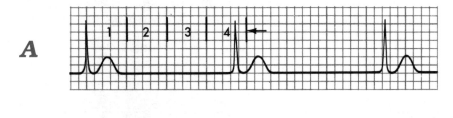

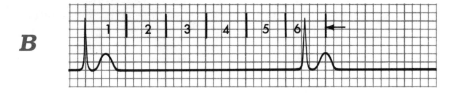

> <u>*Note*</u> → The R-R interval in each example does *not* come out to be an exact number of large boxes.

High Point University
Smith Library
833 Montlieu Ave.
High Point, NC 27262-3598

Answer to Rhythm Strip A:

We are told that the rhythm is regular. The R-R interval measures *between* 3 and 4 large boxes. If it were exactly 3 boxes, the heart rate would be 100 beats/minute (300 ÷ 3); it if were 4 boxes, the heart rate would be 75 beats/minute (300 ÷ 4). Careful inspection suggests that the R-R interval is *closer* to the latter (i.e., to 4 boxes). As a result, we estimate the heart rate to be closer to the *lower* rate number- or *about* **80** beats/minute.

Answer to Rhythm Strip B:

Again we are told that the rhythm is regular. The R-R interval is *between* 5 and 6 large boxes. If it were exactly 5 boxes, the heart rate would be 60 beats/minute (300 ÷ 5); if it were 6 boxes, the heart rate would be 50 beats/minute (300 ÷ 6). Since the R-R interval is approximately *midway* between 5 and 6 large boxes- the heart rate must lie almost midway between 55 and 60 beats/minute- or *about* **55** beats/minute.

Note → Most of the time the R-R interval will *not* be an exact number of large boxes. Use of the process we illustrate above for determining the *relative* position of the R-R interval (with respect to an upper and lower rate limit)- will usually provide a reliable *estimate* of the heart rate.

Calculation of <u>Rate</u>

- When the R-R interval is IRREGULAR -

<u>Question</u> → Why will it be difficult to apply the *'Rule of 300'* to the rhythm shown below? (<u>HINT</u>- *What is happening to the R-R interval?*) Despite this difficulty- *estimate* the heart rate for this example.

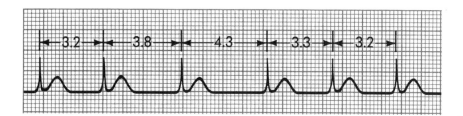

Answer:

It is clearly more difficult to apply the *'Rule of 300'* to the tracing shown on page 51- simply because this rhythm is *NOT* regular. That is, the R-R interval varies in duration from beat to beat. Because most R-R intervals measure *between* 3 and 4 large boxes- we estimate the *heart rate* **range** to be between **75** and **100** beats/minute.

> *Note* → Precise determination of heart rate is impossible when the R-R interval varies- especially when the variation from beat to beat is marked. The most clinically practical way to estimate heart rate in this situation is to provide a **range** within which most R-R intervals will fall.

Calculation of <u>Rate</u>

- When the rhythm is regular and SLOW -

Problem → Calculate the rate for the two examples shown below. Assume in each case that the rhythm is regular.

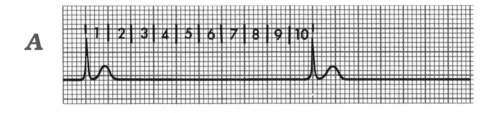

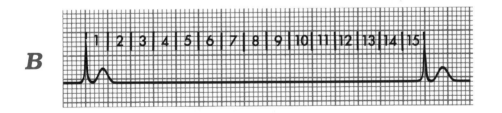

> **Note** → Since we are told that the rhythm is *regular* in each case- we are once again able to use the *'Rule of 300'* to determine the rate.

Answer to Rhythm Strip A:

Only *two* QRS complexes are seen on this tracing. The R-R interval *between* these two complexes counts out to 10 large boxes. In view of this finding, we calculate the heart rate to be $300 \div 10 = $ **30** beats/minute.

Answer to Rhythm Strip B:

Once again, *only* two QRS complexes are seen. The R-R interval between these two complexes counts out to 15 large boxes. Applying the *'Rule of 300'*- we calculate the heart rate to be $300 \div 15 = $ **20** beats/minute.

> **Note** → The beauty of the *'Rule of 300'* is that it works *regardless* of how fast or slow the heart rate happens to be.

Calculation of <u>Rate</u>

- When the rhythm is regular and FAST -

<u>Problem</u> → Calculate the heart rate for the rapid rhythm shown below. *Is the heart rate OVER or UNDER 200 beats/ minute ?*

Lead II

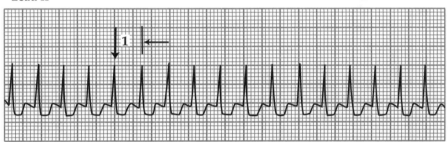

Answer:

The rapid rhythm that is shown on page 55 appears to be regular- which means that we can apply the *'Rule of 300'* to calculate the rate. The first step in this process is to determine the **R-R interval**. This is best done by selecting as a "landmark" an easily recognizable point on a QRS complex that begins or ends on a *heavy* line (*downward arrow on page 55*). Then count over from this point until the next QRS complex.

The R-R interval in this example is between 1 and 2 large boxes. This means that the heart rate must be *between* 150 and 300 beats/minute (*See page 48*). Unfortunately, this rough approximation fails to answer the question we posed as to whether the rate is *over* or *under* 200 beats/minute.

The problem is that when the rhythm is *rapid* and *regular* (as it is here)- even *minor* discrepancies in how one measures the R-R interval may *profoundly* affect the rate you come up with. Use of a simple modification in the *'Rule of 300'*- which we call the **"Every OTHER Beat" Method**- allows you to overcome this difficulty and much more accurately determine the rate: *Simply measure the R-R interval of EVERY OTHER beat.*

Lead II

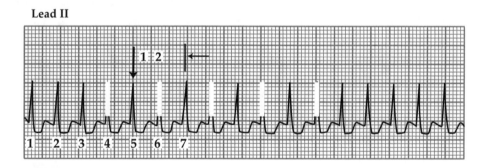

It can now be seen from the above Figure that the R-R interval of every *other* beat is *just under* 3 large boxes. This means that *HALF* the *actual* rate must be *just over* 100- or *about* 105 beats/minute. The *actual* rate for the rhythm on page 55 must therefore be *TWICE* this amount- or *about* **210** beats/minute.

The "<u>*Every OTHER Beat*</u>" *Method*

- Rate calculation when the rhythm is FAST -

<u>Problem</u> → Using the *'Every OTHER Beat' Method*- calculate the heart rate for the rapid rhythm shown below. *Is the heart rate over or under 200 beats/minute?*

Lead II

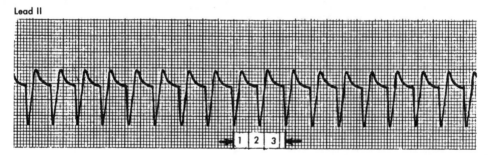

Lead II

Answer:

The rhythm is rapid and regular. The R-R interval is once again *between* 1 and 2 large boxes- which once again means that the heart rate is between 150 and 300 beats/minute. Use of the *'Every OTHER Beat' Method* allows us to determine the rate with much more precision. Thus, it can be seen from the Figure on page 57 that the R-R interval for *every other beat* is a bit over 3 large boxes. This means that *HALF* the rate is ≈85-90 beats/minute. The *actual* rate for this rhythm must therefore be *TWICE* this amount- or *between* **170-180** beats/minute.

In general, heart rate can be rapidly and accurately estimated by using the **'Rule of 300'** (as described on pages 47-48)- especially when the rhythm is regular and the rate is not excessively fast. However- when the rate *IS* fast (*as it is on pages 55 and 57*)- then use of the **"Every OTHER Beat' Method** provides a much more accurate answer.

ECG Terminology

- Use of *Arrhythmia* or *Dysrhythmia* ? -

Question → Which of the above two terms is correct?

Have we used the incorrect term
in the title of this book?

Answer:

Examples of confusing terminology abound in the field of rhythm interpretation. Suffice it to say that on many issues- *NO consensus exists regarding the optimal terminology to use.* The two terms that have probably generated the greatest amount of controversy are *arrhythmia* and *dysrhythmia.* We feel that which one to use is largely a matter of personal preference.

The *purist* undoubtedly favors **dysrhythmia**- despite the fact that this word lacks both the tradition and phonetic facility of arrhythmia. He/she would insist that *arrhythmia* literally means "no rhythm" (or asystole)- since attachment of the prefix "a" to a word implies an "absence of" the entity in question. These individuals prefer to add the prefix "dys" (meaning "a disorder of") to the word stem "rhythm"- and contend that the result- **dys**rhythmia- "properly" connotes a disturbance of rhythm.

We feel this line of reasoning is faulty. In point of fact, the prefix "a" is *not* limited to meaning an "absence of" the entity in question. Instead, it may also be used to imply an *imperfection* of the entity. Furthermore, the root "rhythmos" is *not* restricted to meaning "a regular recurring motion", but instead has also been used to describe "an arrangement, a symmetry, or order"- and *"What could be more disorderly than atrial fibrillation?"* (Marriott, 1984).

Author's Comment → If all words were literally restricted to their derivations and/or original meanings- much of the color and richness of the English language would be lost. Moreover, the *evolutionary* importance accrued from usage over the years would also be lost. We believe the *dictionary* definition of **arrhythmia** (i.e., "a variation from the normal rhythm, especially of the heart beat")- has withstood the test of time. We therefore do *not* ascribe any difference to the meaning of *arrhythmia* and *dysrhythmia*- and we favor using these terms interchangeably. Our personal preference (because of its phonetic facility)- is in favor of the term **arrhythmia**- which is the term we use in all of our written materials.

Systematic Approach
to Arrhythmia Interpretation

- *The 4 Questions* -

(Pages 61 through 86)

> **Note** → The *KEY* to arrhythmia interpretation is to apply a
> **SYSTEMATIC Approach**. In addition to determination of **heart rate** (*See*
> *pages 39-58*)- there are 4 basic points to routinely assess with *every* ECG
> rhythm that is analyzed. We incorporate these points into the
> **4 Questions**- which provide the *framework* for our systematic approach.

Systematic Interpretation- The 4 QUESTION Approach:

Our reason for emphasizing the need to develop a systematic approach to arrhythmia interpretation is *twofold* : 1) It greatly facilitates the process; and 2) It significantly improves accuracy. Even when definitive diagnosis of a particular arrhythmia remains uncertain- *use of a* **SYSTEMATIC Approach** *will* <u>organize thinking</u> *and* <u>narrow</u> *the list of* <u>diagnostic possibilities</u>.

We find that the easiest way to remember the systematic approach is to think of **4 Questions**. Therefore, whenever you are confronted with *any* arrhythmia- *ASK yourself the following* :

- **Question 1**- *Is the rhythm* **REGULAR** ?

- **Question 2**- *Are there* **P waves** ?

- **Question 3**- *Is the* **QRS wide** *or narrow* ?

- **Question 4**- *Is there a* **RELATIONSHIP** *between P waves and the QRS complex* ?

Note → It matters *NOT* in which order you ask yourself these 4 questions. On the contrary- it will often be *preferable* to alter the sequence of these questions (depending on the situation at hand). <u>*What IS important*</u>- *is to ALWAYS include assessment of EACH of these parameters in the analysis of EVERY arrhythmia!*

Use of the
<u>4 QUESTION</u> *Approach*

1) *Is the rhythm* **REGULAR** ?

2)

3)

4)

> **<u>Note</u>** ➔ Many clinicians *intuitively* (and automatically) assess each of the factors included within the *4 Question Approach-* without being aware that they are doing so. We are simply suggesting that *conscious AWARENESS* of the process facilitates interpretation- and makes it much less likely that any important findings will be overlooked.

Question 1 → *Is the Rhythm* **REGULAR** ?

Assessment of **regularity** is usually easy to determine from simple *inspection* of the rhythm. Several points should be kept in mind when evaluating this parameter.

i) In addition to assessing regularity of the *ventricular* response (i.e., of QRS complexes)- it is important to *also* assess regularity of the *atrial* response (i.e., P wave regularity). Although much of the time the pattern of P wave regularity and QRS regularity will be the *same* (because each P wave will be followed by a QRS)- *this will NOT always be the case.*

ii) Assessment of regularity is often a *relative* function. That is, the regularity of any given arrhythmia will often *NOT be* absolute (i.e., either *precisely* regular- or *completely* irregular). Instead, a *gradation* is often present between these two end points on the spectrum (*See page 65 on the* **Patterns** *of* **Regularity**).

iii) Even when the electrical impulse originates as it should from the SA node- there may *normally* be some variation in the regularity of the ventricular response. This is the case with **sinus arrhythmia**- an extremely common *normal* finding in children in which heart rate varies (often markedly) in response to respiration (*See page 95*).

iv) Slight irregularity will often *not* be readily apparent- *unless* P-P and R-R intervals are actually measured. The easiest way to do this is to use **calipers**- which *instantly* reveal even minimal differences in interval duration (*See page 10*). Although much of the time a slight variation in P-P and R-R intervals will *not* be clinically impor- tant- it may sometimes be *very* important!

Patterns of __Regularity__

Clinically- most cardiac rhythms can be described as conforming to one of four general patterns of underlying regularity.

> **__Problem__** → For each of the 4 schematic patterns that are shown below, indicate whether the pattern is *precisely* regular- *almost* regular- or clearly *NOT regular*. If the pattern is *not* regular- indicate whether there is a sense of *group beating* (i.e., a *"regular irregularity"*) to the pattern- or whether complexes in the pattern appear to occur in completely *random* fashion.

Answer:

It will usually be *surprisingly EASY* to classify the regularity of most cardiac rhythms into one of the 4 general patterns that are shown the preceding page:

- **Pattern 1-** which is *completely* **regular** (i.e., *without* demonstrable variation in the interval between one complex and the next).

- **Pattern 2-** which is *fairly* **regular** (i.e., with only *minimal* variation in the interval between one complex and the next). Differentiation between this pattern and Pattern 1 may sometimes be difficult (unless the interval between complexes is are carefully measured).

- **Pattern 3-** which is *regularly* **irregular** (i.e., with the phenomenon of *"group beating"*- in which complexes are *grouped* into a *regularly* repetitive pattern).

- **Pattern 4-** which is *completely* **irregular** (i.e., with continual *random* and *unpredictable* variation in the interval between complexes- so that there is *NO semblance* of any organized pattern).

> **Note** → Practically speaking- it will often be easiest to determine the overall pattern of rhythm regularity by *stepping back* a short distance from the tracing being examined. This is especially true with regard to recognizing the "group beating" pattern of *regular irregularity* (Pattern 3 above). For this reason, it is sometimes said that the phenomenon of **group beating** is appreciated best *"from the back of the room"* (i.e., at a distance *away* from the tracing being examined).

Early and Late Beats

In addition to the overall patterns of rhythm regularity (described on pages 65-66)- unexpectedly *EARLY* or *LATE* beats may occur that alter the underlying pattern of the general rhythm. The appearance and *timing* of such beats provide invaluable clues to their etiology.

Problem → Examine the three patterns of rhythm regularity that are shown below. The rhythm is *completely* regular in Pattern 1. Beats **X** and **Y** (in Patterns 5 and 6) interrupt what otherwise would also be regular patterns. *Do beats X and Y occur EARLY or LATE ?*

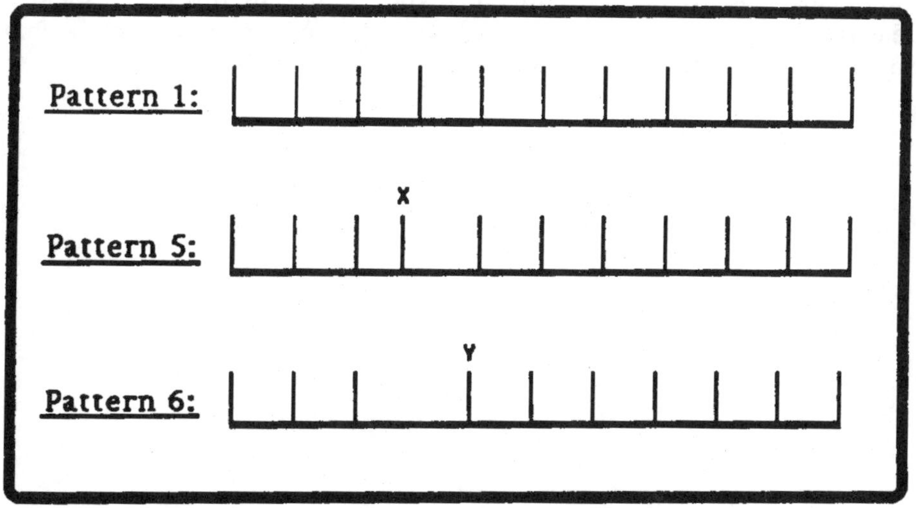

Answer:

As noted, **Pattern 1** is *completely regular.* There is *NO variation* in the interval between any one complex and the next (*page 65*). In contrast, the regularity of the other two patterns is interrupted in each case by the 4th beat:

- **Pattern 5**- in which the 4th beat (labeled **X**) occurs *EARLY* (i.e., is *"premature"*). As discussed on page 16- ***premature* beats** may originate from one of 3 possible sites: 1) from elsewhere in the *atria* (i.e., **PACs**); 2) from within the *AV node* (i.e., **PJCs**); or 3) from somewhere in the *ventricles* (i.e., **PVCs**).

- **Pattern 6**- in which the 4th beat (labeled **Y**) occurs *LATE.* Late-occurring beats are perhaps best thought of as ***"escape"* beats**. By definition, their appearance is *delayed* until *after* the failure of the dominant pacemaker. These beats serve as *rescue* beats- that arise (i.e., *"escape"*) in an effort to prevent excessive slowing of the underlying rhythm. As implied by their name, *escape* (or *"rescue"*) beats may be extremely beneficial- especially when they appear in response to what otherwise might be a life-threatening bradycardia.

Recognizing the Patterns

- **Practice** -

Examine the 2 rhythms that are shown below. *Focus on the QRS complexes.* Which of the 6 patterns of **rhythm regularity** (discussed on pages 65-68) best describes each example? *What other observations can you make ?*

A

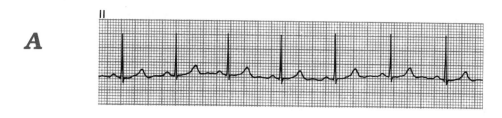

B

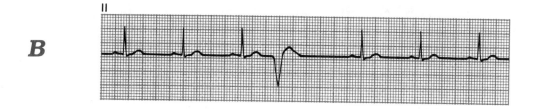

Answer to Example A:

The rhythm is *completely* regular- since there is no variation in the R-R interval between one QRS complex and the next. This example corresponds to **Pattern 1** that was shown on page 65.

> Looking closer at the rhythm, it can be seen that *all* 3 of the essential components of an ECG complex (i.e., **P** wave, **QRS** complex, and **T** wave- *See page 17*) are present with each beat. Note in particular that the P wave preceding each QRS complex appears to be *related* to that QRS (i.e., the PR interval appears to be constant). This is a ***normal sinus rhythm (NSR)***. By the *'Rule of 300'*- we estimate the heart rate to be approximately 75 beats/minute (since the R-R interval is about 4 large boxes in duration).

Answer to Example B:

In contrast to Example A, this rhythm is *not* completely regular. Instead, it is interrupted by an *early* occurring beat. This example corresponds to **Pattern 5** that was shown on page 67.

> With the exception of the early occurring beat, it can be seen that the *underlying* rhythm is really quite regular. Looking closer at this *early* beat- one should strongly suspect it to be arising from a site in the ventricles (i.e., to be a **PVC**)- because it is *wide* and looks so *different* from the normally conducted sinus beats (*See page 15*).

Recognizing the Patterns

- **Practice** (Continued) -

Examine the 2 rhythms that are shown below. *Focus on the QRS complexes.* Which of the 6 patterns of **rhythm regularity** (discussed on page 65-68) best describes each example? *What other observations can you make?*

C

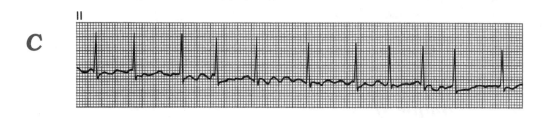

D

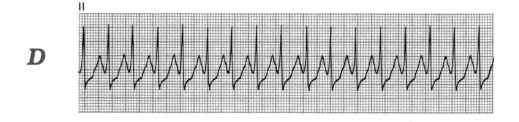

Answer to Example C:

The rhythm is completely *irregular*- since there is *continual* (and *unpredictable*) variation in the R-R interval from one QRS complex to the next. This example corresponds to **Pattern 4** that was shown on page 65.

> Looking closer at this rhythm, it can be seen that although there are undulations in the baseline- there is *no definite P wave* in front of the QRS complexes. This rhythm is **atrial fibrillation** (which *will* be discussed in detail *on pages 103-108*). Because the R-R interval continually varies, we can't determine an exact rate- but instead can estimate a *heart rate* **range** (*See pages 51-52*). Since most R-R intervals are *between* 2.5 to 4 large boxes in duration- the heart rate varies between 75 to 120 beats/minute.

Answer to Example D:

This rhythm *is* completely regular- albeit at an extremely rapid rate. It corresponds to **Pattern 1** that was shown on page 65.

> The R-R interval is between 1 and 2 large boxes in duration. When the rhythm is this fast, we favor use of the *'Every OTHER Beat' Method* to calculate the rate (*See pages 55-58*). Since the heart rate for every *other* beat (i.e., *HALF* the rate) is about 85 beats/minute- the *actual* rate should be *twice* this amount- or about 170 beats/minute.
>
> Regarding other observations about this rhythm- it is difficult to be sure if the pointed upright deflections that appear between QRS complexes are P waves- T waves- or both. As one might imagine- *it will therefore be difficult to determine with certainty the etiology of this arrhythmia.*

Use of the
<u>4 QUESTION</u> *Approach*

1)

2) *Are there* **P waves** ?

3)

4)

<u>Note</u> → It may already be apparent that even though we list the search for P waves as a *separate* question- *EACH of the 4 Questions are closely interrelated with each other.*

Question 2 → *Are there **P waves**?*

Detection of **P waves** is really the cornerstone of arrhythmia interpretation. When the rhythm is sinus- the process is easy (because P waves *regularly* occur before QRS complexes- *See Example A on page 69*). At other times, detection of P waves may be much more difficult (*See Example D on page 71*).

The *KEY* point to emphasize is that *by definition*- the **P wave** should *ALWAYS* be **upright** in standard **lead II** with ***normal sinus rhythm***. This is because orientation of the electrical impulse as it travels from the SA node to the AV node (*arrow in the Figure below*) is virtually *parallel* to lead II. Therefore- <u>IF</u> the electrical impulse originates from the SA node- and travels over the normal conduction pathway (i.e., toward the AV node)- it should be viewed as *approaching* (and inscribe a *positive* or *upright* P wave) in standard lead II.

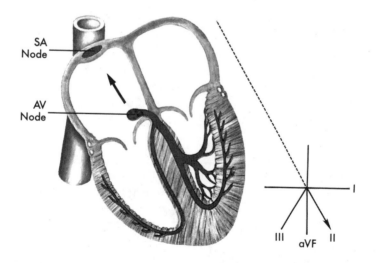

P Wave Polarity in Lead II

We emphasized on page 74 that the P wave should *always* be upright in standard lead II when the rhythm is sinus.

Lead II

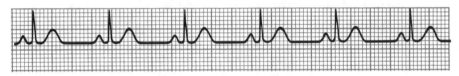

Normal Sinus Rhythm

Problem → There are 2 *exceptions* to the above statement (i.e., in which the P wave will *not* be upright *despite* the fact that the patient is in sinus rhythm). *Can you think of what they are?*

HINT- The above statement assumes a normal anatomic location for the heart (i.e., on the *left* side of the chest)- and also assumes that technical aspects of the recording (i.e., lead placement, etc.) have all been properly attended to.

Answer:

If the rhythm is **sinus**- then the P wave should be *upright* in lead II. The *only* exceptions to this rule are:

> i) If the patient has *dextrocardia*.
> ii) If the leads are reversed.

In clinical practice, *lead reversal* is by far the more common occurrence of the two. Fortunately (for rhythm analysis purposes)- *both* of these clinical situations are uncommon. Therefore- for practical purposes it will usually be safe to assume the following:

> If P waves are *not* upright in lead II- *the mechanism of the rhythm is NOT sinus.*

Note → Return for a moment to pages 27-28- in which we discussed the most commonly preferred **monitoring leads**. It should now be clear that the major benefits of using **lead II** as a monitoring lead are that it provides an excellent view of atrial activity- and that it allows you to tell in an instant if the rhythm is sinus- *simply by looking to see if the P wave is upright in this lead.*

Is the Rhythm Sinus?

- Practice -

Examine the rhythm that is shown below. Note that it was obtained from a lead II monitoring lead. *Is it likely that the rhythm is sinus?*

Lead II

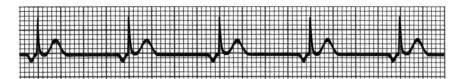

Answer:

No. It is highly *unlikely* that the rhythm on the preceding page is sinus- *because the P wave is NOT upright in lead II.* The only possible way in which this rhythm could represent a sinus-initiated mechanism would be:

i) If the patient had dextrocardia

and/or

ii) If the leads were reversed.

As emphasized on page 76- for practical purposes (i.e., assuming that the patient does *not* have dextrocardia or lead reversal)- it can be said that:

> If P waves are *not* upright in lead II- *the mechanism of the rhythm is NOT sinus.*

Note → As we will soon discuss, the mechanism of the rhythm that appears on page 77 is *junctional* (i.e., *AV nodal* rhythm)- in which the "pacemak-ing" site of the heart has shifted from the SA node to the AV node (which accounts for the *negative* P wave that is seen in lead II).

Use of the
<u>4 QUESTION</u> *Approach*

1)

2)

3) *Is the* **QRS wide** *or narrow ?*

4)

KEY → Normally in adults- the process of ventricular depolarization (as described on pages 13-14) is complete in *no more* than 0.10 second. As a result, the QRS complex will normally be inscribed *within* this period of time. The QRS complex is said to be **WIDE** if it takes *longer* than this (i.e., if it takes **more** than **0.10 second** in duration). Since one *large* box on ECG grid paper corresponds to a period of 0.20 second (*See page 37*)- one can tell at a glance if the QRS is wide- *simply by looking to see if the QRS complex is* **more** *than* **HALF** *a* **large box** *in duration.*

Question 3 → *Is the QRS wide or narrow ?*

Evaluation of the **width** of the **QRS complex** is a *KEY* parameter for determining the site of origin of the electrical impulse:

- IF the QRS complex is of **normal duration** (i.e., *NOT* more than *half* a large box in duration)- then the electrical impulse will almost certainly be of *SUPRAventricular* etiology (i.e., originating from a site that is either at or above the *double dotted line* in the Figure below).

- *In contrast*- IF the QRS complex is **WIDE** (i.e., *more* than *half* a large box in duration- or *at least* 0.11 second)- then the electrical impulse is likely to be of *VENTRICULAR* origin- although (as discussed on pages 21-22) it still *could* be supraventricular- *IF* there is a *bundle branch block* or *aberrant conduction.*

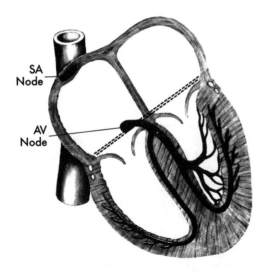

The **double dotted line** in the Figure delineates the boundary that separates the atria from the ventricles. Beats or rhythms that originate *at* or *above* the double dotted line are termed **SUPRAventricular**- because their site of origin is *above* (i.e., "*SUPRA*" to) the ventricles. This includes impulses that originate from the SA node, from elsewhere in one of the atria- and/or from the AV node itself. Ventricular beats or rhythms originate from a site *below* the line.

Is the QRS Wide or Narrow ?

- **Practice** -

Examine the 2 ECG complexes that are shown below. *Is the QRS wide or narrow ?*

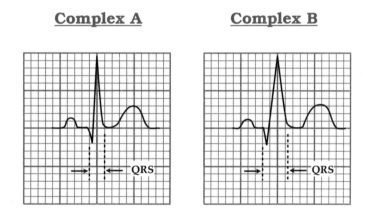

Complex A   ### Complex B

HINT- In formulating your answer- remember the dimensions of ECG grid paper that were introduced on page 37 (i.e., **0.04 second** for a **small box**; and **0.20 second** for a **large box**). Keep in mind that *normal* duration for the QRS complex in adults is *up to* (and *including*) 0.10 second.

Answer:

It can be seen from the Figure on the preceding page that the QRS interval of **Complex A** is 2 *little* boxes in duration. This comes out to a QRS interval of **0.08 second** (i.e., 0.04 second X 2 little boxes = 0.08)- which is clearly *within* the normal range for QRS duration. Thus, the QRS of Complex A is said to be **narrow**.

In contrast- the QRS interval of **Complex B** is *more* than 3 little boxes in duration. This corresponds to a QRS interval of about **0.14 second**- which is clearly prolonged and qualifies Complex B to be described as **wide**.

Note → The more leads available for monitoring- the more accurate assessment of QRS interval duration will be (*See page 10*). This is because sometimes a portion of the QRS complex may lie on the baseline- in which case one may get the false impression from viewing a particular lead that the QRS complex is *narrower* than it really is. Assuming the patient is hemodynamically stable- one should ideally consider use of *more* than a single monitoring lead (and/or obtaining a 12-lead ECG)- whenever this is clinically possible.

Use of the
4 QUESTION Approach

1)

2)

3)

4) *Is there a* **RELATIONSHIP** *between*
  P waves and the QRS complex ?

Note → This 4th Question is *easy* to answer when the rhythm is sinus and P waves are ***"married"*** to the QRS complex. However, when P waves are present but the mechanism of the rhythm is something *other than* normal sinus rhythm- answering this question may become much more difficult. This is especially true when the number of P waves and QRS complexes is *not* equal (i.e., when AV conduction is *not* 1:1).

Question 4 → *Is there a RELATIONSHIP between P waves and the QRS complex?*

P waves are *not* always present in every arrhythmia. When P waves are absent- it should be apparent that this 4th Question *cannot* be addressed.

When P waves are present (as they will be in *most* arrhythmias- the *KEY* to interpretation will lie with determining the **relationship** (if any) between P waves and the QRS complex. In clinical practice, the most common "relationship" (*by far* !) is the one that is seen with **normal sinus rhythm (NSR)**- in which a P wave is present for *each* QRS complex. In this relationship, *each* P wave is *conducted* to the ventricles (*See Example A on page 69*). The result is a PR interval that is *fixed* (i.e., *constant*)- so that it appears as if each P wave is **"married"** to its respective QRS.

The relationship that occurs with NSR between P waves and their respective QRS complex is described as **1:1 AV conduction**. That is- *one* **A**trial-initiated impulse (i.e., *one* P wave)- is present for every *one* QRS (i.e., **V**entricular) complex. By way of comparison, with 2:1 AV block (*which we will discuss in Section 1G beginning on page 235*)- there are *two* P waves for every QRS. Other AV conduction ratios (i.e., 3:1, 3:2, 4:1, etc.)- as well as *other* relationships (i.e., the progressively *lengthening* PR interval of Wenckebach block) are possible.

Suggested Approach → To determine if P waves are **related** to the QRS complex (and if so- *HOW*)- we find it easiest to *FIRST* focus on simply *identifying* all QRS complexes on the tracing. Then look *in front* of each QRS to see if a P wave is present- and if so, determine the PR interval. Survey the entire tracing to see if this PR interval changes- or if it remains the same for all beats on the tracing (as it will when the P waves are **"married"**). Finally- account for any P waves that may *not* be followed by a QRS (i.e., for any P waves that may *not* be conducted).

Putting It All Together

- Applying the 4 Question Approach -

Examine the rhythm below *putting together* the concepts that we have incorporated into the **4 Question Approach**. (Feel free to refer to pages 61 through 84 in formulating your answer.)

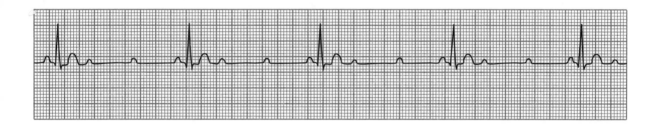

Note → As emphasized on page 62- the *sequence* for assessing the parameters contained within the 4 Questions may be freely *altered*. Our preference is to begin with *whichever* parameter is *easiest* to evaluate for the particular arrhythmia- be this regularity of the rhythm, identification of P waves, or determination of QRS width.

HINT- Consider use of the **Suggested Approach** described on page 84 when attempting to answer the 4th Question (which addresses the *relationship* between P waves and the QRS complex).

Answer:

Applying the **4 Question Approach** to the rhythm that appears on the front of this card (and *labeling* our observations in the Figure below)- we note the following:

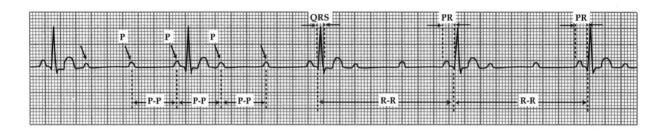

i) P waves *are* present throughout the tracing (*Question 2*).

ii) The QRS complex appears to be *narrow* (i.e., the QRS is *NOT more* than *half* a large box in duration). This implies that the *mechanism* of the rhythm must be *SUPRAventricular* (*Question 3*).

iii) The rhythm is *regular* (*Question 1*). This holds true for *both* the P wave rhythm (i.e., the P-P interval is constant)- as well as for the ventricular rhythm (since the R-R interval is also constant). The P-P interval is slightly *less* than 3 large boxes in duration- which corresponds to an *atrial* rate of about 105 beats/minute. The R-R interval is between 8 to 9 large boxes in duration- which corresponds to a *ventricular* rate of about 35 beats/minute.

iv) There *is* a relation between P waves and the QRS complex (*Question 4*). Thus, it can be seen that *each* QRS in the tracing *is* preceded by a P wave- and that the PR interval preceding each QRS is *fixed* (i.e., constant). However- *NOT* all P waves are *followed* by a QRS- so that *only* 1 out of 3 P waves is conducted to the ventricles (i.e., there is 3:1 AV conduction).

Section 1C- *SUPRAVentricular* **Rhythms**

Basic Rhythms

Armed with the knowledge we presented in <u>Section 1A</u> on ***Introductory Concepts***- and in <u>Section 1B</u> on the systematic ***4 Question Approach***- virtually *any* cardiac arrhythmia can now be evaluated.

The *framework* from which we develop our system for classifying the basic cardiac arrhythmias is shown below. Practically speaking, the number of *basic rhythms* that need to be mastered is limited (See page 88). Simple awareness of the most common arrhythmias that are likely to be encountered in clinical practice will go a surprisingly long way toward facilitating diagnosis.

Most arrhythmias can be categorized into one of the following 5 groups:

1. ***Sinus Mechanism Rhythms/Arrhythmias***

2. ***Other SUPRAVentricular Arrhythmias***

3. ***Premature Beats***

4. ***Sustained Ventricular Arrhythmias***

5. ***AV Blocks***

The Basic Rhythms

1. ## Sinus Mechanism Rhythms/Arrhythmias
   - Normal sinus rhythm (NSR)
   - Sinus bradycardia
   - Sinus tachycardia
   - Sinus arrhythmia

2. ## Other SupraVentricular Arrhythmias
   - Atrial fibrillation
     - MAT (multifocal atrial tachycardia)
   - Atrial flutter
   - PSVT (paroxysmal supraventricular tachycardia)
   - Junctional (AV nodal) rhythms:
     - AV nodal *escape* rhythm
     - Accelerated junctional rhythm
     - Junctional tachycardia

3. ## Premature Beats
   - PACs (premature *atrial* contractions)
   - PJCs (premature *junctional* contractions)
   - PVCs (premature *ventricular* contractions)

4. ## Sustained Ventricular Arrhythmias
   - Idioventricular *escape* rhythm
   - AIVR (accelerated idioventricular escape rhythm)
   - Ventricular tachycardia
   - Ventricular fibrillation

5. ## AV Blocks

SINUS Mechanism
Rhythms

As emphasized on pages 73-76- **SINUS-mechanism rhythms** are defined by the presence of an *upright* P wave in standard lead II.

Lead II

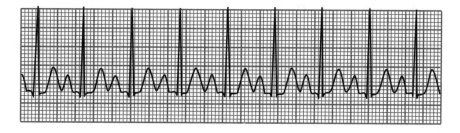

The Common SINUS-Mechanism Rhythms:

1. Normal sinus rhythm (NSR)
2. Sinus bradycardia
3. Sinus tachycardia
4. Sinus arrhythmia

Recognition:

As illustrated by the tracing page 89- a **SINUS-*mechanism* rhythm** is readily recognized by the presence of *upright* P waves in standard lead II that *consistently* precede each QRS complex. The PR interval should be *constant* (i.e., *fixed*) and of *normal* duration- unless some type of AV block is present. Note that P wave morphology stays the same for *all* P waves on the tracing that appears page 89- supporting the notion that each atrial impulse originates from the *same* site (which in this case *by definition* is the SA node).

The Common SINUS-Mechanism Rhythms:

1. **Normal sinus rhythm (NSR)**- regular rhythm; rate *between* 60-99 beats/minute.

2. **Sinus bradycardia**- regular rhythm; rate *below* 60 beats/ minute (*See page 93*).

3. **Sinus tachycardia**- regular rhythm; rate *above* 99 beats/ minute (*as is the case for the rhythm page 89*).

4. **Sinus arrhythmia**- *irregular* rhythm despite the presence of a sinus mechanism (*See page 95*).

Note → Although the P wave *must* be upright in standard lead II for the rhythm to be sinus (assuming no dextrocardia or lead reversal)- this is *not* necessarily true for other monitoring leads. For example, P waves may *either* be upright *or* negative with sinus rhythm when MCL_1 is the lead that is used for monitoring.

Is the Rhythm Sinus?

The 12-lead ECG shown below was obtained from a patient with acute inferior infarction. *What is the rhythm?*

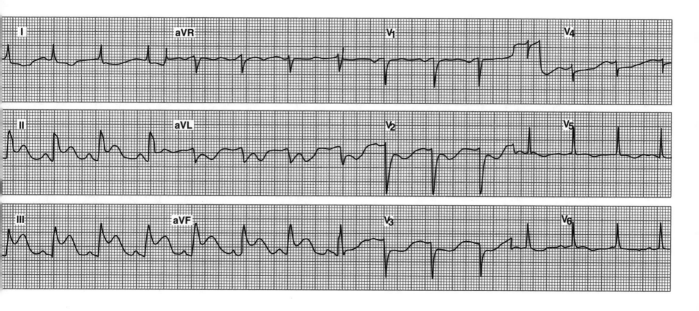

KEY Point → Which is the *BEST* lead to look at for determining the rhythm on a 12-lead ECG? Note the appearance of the P wave in *this* particular lead- *as well as in each of the other 11 leads on the tracing.*

Answer:

The *BEST* lead to look at for determining the rhythm on a 12-lead ECG is standard **lead II**. This is because- *by definition*- the **P wave** should always be ***upright*** in this lead if the rhythm is **sinus**. Note that the P wave *IS* upright in lead II of this 12-lead ECG (*solid arrows below*).

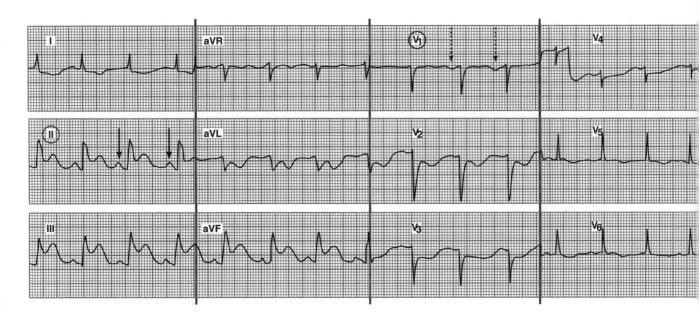

> ***Note*** → P waves are *not* nearly as well seen in other leads on this ECG. Note in particular that *despite* the presence of normal sinus rhythm (as determined by the presence of *upright* P waves in lead II)- P waves are *not* necessarily upright in *other* leads on the tracing (i.e., *broken arrows in lead V$_1$*).

Sinus *Bradycardia*

Lead II

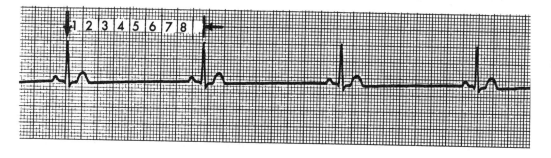

Question → What is the *clinical* significance of the rhythm shown above? Despite the slow rate- *can you think of a situation in which this rhythm might be normal*?

Interpretation:

Applying the **4 *Question Approach*** to the rhythm that appears on page 93- we note the following:

    i) *P waves* are present. They are *upright* in this lead II monitoring lead- which means that there is a **sinus** mechanism.

    ii) The QRS complex is *narrow* (i.e., it is *not more* than *half* a large box in duration).

    iii) The rhythm is *regular*- albeit exceedingly slow. The R-R interval is between 8 and 9 large boxes. If it were 8 boxes- the heart rate would be 38 beats/minute (i.e., $300 \div 8$). If it were 10 boxes- the rate would be 30 beats/minute (i.e., $300 \div 10$). We therefore estimate the rate to be *about* **35 beats/minute**.

    iv) Despite the slow rate- P waves *are* related to the QRS complex. This is apparent from the fact that *each* QRS *is* preceded by a P wave- and the PR interval is *fixed* (i.e., *all* P waves are *"married"* to their respective QRS). This is as it should be when the rhythm is sinus. Since the heart rate is *less* than 60 beats/minute, the rhythm is **Sinus Bradycardia**.

Clinical Notes ➔ The significance of sinus bradycardia depends on the clinical setting in which it occurs. Marked sinus bradycardia (i.e., to the extent that is shown on page 93) is clearly of concern when it occurs in the setting of acute myocardial infarction or cardiopulmonary arrest. On the other hand, resting sinus bradycardia with a heart rate between 30-40 beats/minute might be a perfectly *normal* finding for an asymptomatic, otherwise healthy long-distance runner in peak condition.

Sinus <u>Arrhythmia</u>

Lead II

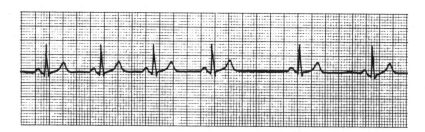

Question → What is the *clinical* significance of the rhythm shown above? When will you most commonly see this rhythm?

Interpretation:

Applying the **4 *Question Approach*** to the rhythm that appears on page 95- we note the following:

i) *P waves* are present. They are *upright* in this lead II monitoring lead- which means that there is a **sinus** mechanism.

ii) Despite the presence of a sinus mechanism- the rhythm is clearly *not* regular (i.e., R-R intervals obviously vary from one beat to the next). Since most R-R intervals look to be *between* 4 and 6 large boxes in duration- we estimate the **heart rate range** to be *between* 50-75 beats/minute.

iii) The QRS complex is *narrow* (i.e., it is *not more* than *half* a large box in duration).

iv) Despite irregularity of the rhythm- P waves *are* related to the QRS complex. That is, *each* QRS complex *is* preceded by a P wave- and the PR interval is *fixed* (i.e., *all* P waves on the tracing are "*married*" to their respective QRS). Thus, we interpret this rhythm as **Sinus Arrhythmia**.

Clinical Notes → As with *all* sinus mechanism rhythms- the significance of sinus arrhythmia depends on the clinical setting in which it occurs. Sinus arrhythmia is an exceedingly common *normal* finding in otherwise healthy, asymptomatic children and young adults- in whom the rhythm will often vary according to the phase of respiration. In contrast, marked sinus arrhythmia may be a pathologic finding if it occurs in an older patient with symptoms of syncope (for whom the rhythm may be a manifestation of sick sinus syndrome).

Sinus <u>Tachycardia</u>

Lead II

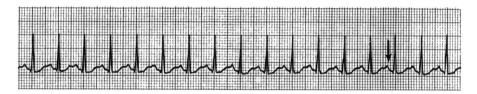

<u>Question</u> → What is the *clinical* significance of the rhythm shown above? *How certain should you be that this rhythm is truly sinus tachycardia?*

Interpretation:

Applying the *4 Question Approach* to the rhythm that appears on page 97- we note the following:

i) The rhythm is *regular*- and fast. The R-R interval is 2 large boxes in duration- which means that the rate is **150 beats/minute** (i.e., 300 ÷ 2).

ii) The QRS complex is *narrow* (i.e., it is clearly *not more* than *half* a large box in duration). The rhythm is therefore *SUPRAventricular.*

iii) & iv) The presence (and nature) of P waves on this tracing is uncertain. Although it appears that P waves precede each QRS complex (*arrow*)- and that P waves are *"married"* to the QRS with a *fixed* PR interval- the rapidity of the rate makes it difficult to be certain that these deflections *truly* are P waves (and not just the terminal portion of the ST segment and T wave). Without additional information (i.e., additional leads)- it may *not* be possible to render a *definitive* diagnosis. We therefore qualify our interpretation as <u>*probable*</u> **Sinus Tachycardia** (pending confirmation that these deflections *truly* are P waves).

<u>Clinical Notes</u> → As illustrated by this example, a problem that may be encountered with sinus tachycardia when the rate is rapid- is that P waves may *blend* with T waves- and *definitive diagnosis may not be possible.* Clinically- it is helpful to remember that sinus tachycardia **rarely exceeds 150-160 beats/minute** (or *at most* 170 beats/minute) in a *"horizontal"* (i.e., hospitalized) *adult.* Faster rates may be seen with sinus tachycardia in children- and/or in adults who are exercising. In other situations- the finding of a tachycardia with a heart rate that is *greater* than 160-170 beats/minute makes it highly *unlikely* that the rhythm is sinus tachycardia.

The point to emphasize about management of sinus tachycardia is that the treatment of choice is to determine and correct the *underlying* cause- and *not* to treat the rhythm per se.

Practice: *What is the rhythm?*

Lead MCL₁

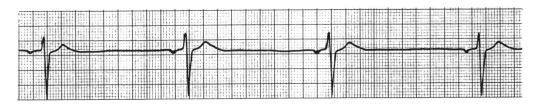

Question → Despite the fact that P waves are *not* upright in the above tracing- *could the rhythm be sinus* ?

HINT- Feel free to refer to our **Note** on page 90.

Interpretation:

Applying the **4 Question Approach** to the rhythm that appears on page 99- we note the following:

i) The rhythm appears to be *fairly* regular. However, it is *NOT completely regular-* as the R-R interval for the last beat on the tracing *is* longer (by about 3 little boxes) than the R-R interval of the first two beats. Since R-R intervals are *between* 10 and 11 large boxes in duration- we estimate the heart rate to be *about* **30 beats/minute**.

ii) The QRS complex appears to be at the upper limit of normal (i.e., it is *about* half a large box in duration).

iii) & iv) P waves *are* present. They appear as small *negative* deflections that precede each QRS complex with a *fixed* PR interval in this MCL_1 monitoring lead. Thus, each P wave *is* "married" to its respective QRS. The mechanism is therefore presumed to be *sinus-* and we describe the rhythm as *marked* **Sinus Bradycardia** and **Arrhythmia**.

Note → It will sometimes be difficult to distinguish between the slight (and acceptable) degree of variability that is commonly seen with normal sinus rhythm (NSR)- and the somewhat greater degree of irregularity that characterizes sinus "arrhythmia". Fortunately, distinction between these two entities is usually academic- since the clinical significance of sinus arrhythmia *rarely* differs from the clinical signficance of NSR.

Technically speaking- a sinus mechanism rhythm is classified as **sinus "arrhythmia"-** when the degree of variability of R-R intervals *exceeds* 2 to 3 little boxes (i.e., is *greater* than 0.08- 0.12 second). This is the case for the rhythm that appears on page 99- as well as for the rhythm that appears on page 95.

Other <u>**SUPRAVentricular**</u>
(i.e., NARROW QRS) **Rhythms**

As emphasized on page 80- ***SUPRAventricular rhythms*** are those in which the electrical impluse originates *at* or *above* the AV node (i.e., at or above the *double dotted line* in the Figure below):

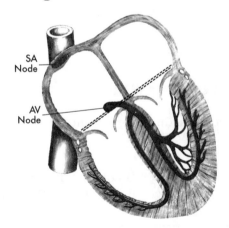

<u>*The Most Common SUPRA-Ventricular Rhythms*</u>:

> 1. Sinus Mechanism Rhythms
> 2. Atrial fibrillation
> 3. Atrial flutter
> 4. PSVT (paroxysmal supraventricular tachycardia)
> 5. Junctional (AV nodal) rhythms

Recognition:

By definition- ***SUPRA-Ventricular rhythms*** originate *at* or *above* the AV node (i.e., at or above the *double dotted line* in the Figure on page 101). In addition to the **sinus mechanism rhythms** that were just discussed (*See pages 89-100*)- the other principal entities in this category include:

- **Atrial fibrillation** (*See pages 103-110*)

- **Atrial flutter** (*See pages 111-124*)

- **PSVT** (*See pages 125-132*)

- **Junctional (AV nodal) rhythms** (*See pages 141-150*)

The clinical point to emphasize regarding the *origination* site of any cardiac arrhythmia relates to the importance of determining QRS width:

> If you can be *certain* that the QRS complex is *truly NARROW* (i.e., in *all* 12 leads)- then for all practical purposes- *the rhythm MUST be SUPRAventricular.*

KEY→ Once established that a particular rhythm is of *SUPRAventricular* etiology- diagnosis of the *specific* type of supraventricular rhythm can then be made based on calculation of *heart rate*- and attention to the remaining items of our *4 Question Approach* (i.e., *regularity* of the rhythm- identification of *P waves* or other evidence of atrial activity- and the *relation*, if any, of such P waves to the QRS).

Atrial Fibrillation

Use the **4 *Question* Approach** to interpret the rhythm shown below.

Lead II

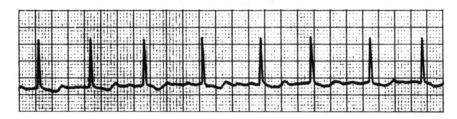

KEY Questions:

1. Describe the *pattern of regularity* for the above rhythm. (Feel free to refer to page 65 in formulating your answer.)

   HINT- You may want to *measure* all R-R intervals (ideally with **calipers**)- *BEFORE* committing yourself to an answer.

2. Do you see evidence of *atrial* activity?

Interpretation:

Applying the _**4 Question Approach**_ to the rhythm that appears on page 103- we note the following:

i) The QRS complex is _narrow_ (i.e., clearly _not more_ than _half_ a large box in duration). This means that the rhythm must be _SUPRAventricular_- and is likely to be one of the entities listed on page 101.

ii) _P waves are absent._ This essentially _rules out_ a sinus mechanism rhythm (because a definite upright P wave should always be seen in lead II if the rhythm is sinus).

iii) The rhythm is _irregularly irregular._ Although the amount of variability between one R-R interval and the next is _not_ great- the R-R interval _does_ vary from one beat to the next (i.e., the pattern of regularity corresponds to **Pattern 4** on page 65).

> **Comment** → The rhythm that appears on the front of this card is _supraventricular_ (because the QRS is narrow)- _irregularly irregular_- and _without_ P waves. These findings comprise the clinical definition of _**Atrial Fibrillation (A Fib)**_- in this case with a _**controlled**_ ventricular response.

> **Note** → We are only able to address 3 of the 4 Questions of our _Systematic Approach_ for this arrhythmia. There is no need to look for a _relation_ between "P waves" and the QRS complex- _because there are no P waves._
>
> _Instead of P waves_- there are fine undulations in the baseline. These undulations most likely represent _**"fib waves"**_- that reflect the chaotic activity of atria that are fibrillating at an exceedingly rapid rate (that usually exceeds 400 times per minute). Sometimes fib waves are obvious (i.e., "coarse"- and of large amplitude). At other times, they are much less readily apparent (as is the case here).

Atrial Fibrillation

- The *Ventricular* Response -

Simply interpreting a rhythm as "atrial fibrillation" is an *incomplete* description. Mention should *also* be made of the ventricular response- which reflects the *average* ventricular rate. Optimal interpretation of **Atrial Fibrillation** would therefore include one of the three following descriptors:

- A Fib with a **RAPID** *ventricular response*

- A Fib with a **controlled** (or **moderate**) *ventricular response*

- A Fib with a **SLOW** *ventricular response*

Clinical Note → As discussed on page 104, the chaotic activity of fibrillating atria will often produce irregularly occurring **"fib waves"** that disturb the isoelectric ECG baseline. These fib waves may be **"coarse"** (i.e., of large amplitude)- or they may be **"fine"** and barely visible (if seen at all). As might be imagined, identification of A Fib may become much more difficult when fib waves are barely detectable- in which case the diagnosis will have to depend on recognition of an *irregularly irregular* rhythm- and the *absence* of P waves anywhere on the tracing.

II

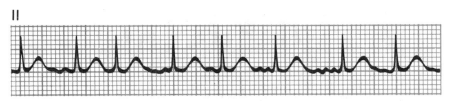

- ▪ *A **Fib** with a **RAPID** ventricular response*- in which heart rate averages *over* 120 beats/minute (i.e., most R-R intervals are *between* 2 to 3 large boxes in duration). Note that fib waves on this tracing are barely detectable.

II

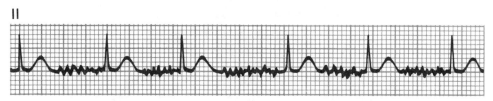

- ▪ *A **Fib** with a **CONTROLLED** ventricular response*- in which heart rate averages *between* 70-110 beats/minute (i.e., most R-R intervals are *between* 3 large boxes or a little less- and 4 large boxes or a little more in duration). The **fib waves** in this example are "coarse".

II

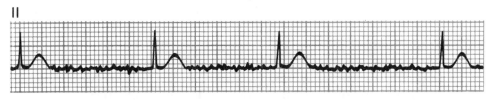

- ▪ *A **Fib** with a **SLOW** ventricular response*- in which heart rate averages *less* than 60 beats/minute (i.e., most R-R intervals are *more* than 5 large boxes in duration). The **fib waves** in this example are "fine".

Atrial Fibrillation

- Clinical Significance -

In patients with an otherwise normal heart, the abrupt onset of A Fib will usually be accompanied by a *rapid* ventricular response.

II

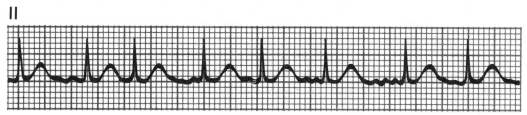

Clinically- *three* major consequences may result from development of A Fib. These include:

1. Symptoms (as sensed by the patient- usually in the form of palpitations).
2. An increased risk of thromboembolism (as a result of the stasis produced by *noncontractile* fibrillating atria).
3. Hemodynamic compromise (in the form of heart failure, pulmonary edema, hypotension).

Question → Why is new-onset A Fib so commonly associated with development of heart failure- especially in elderly patients?

HINT- What happens to the *"atrial kick"* with A Fib? What happens to the time available for *diastolic filling* of the ventricles?

Answer:

Heart failure commonly develops in patients with new-onset A Fib as a result of two factors: 1) Loss of the *"atrial kick"* ; and 2) Reduced ventricular filling during the period of diastole.

Many elderly patients who have only marginal ventricular function become very dependent on the 5-40% contribution to cardiac output that atrial contraction provides. This contraction is entirely lost with the loss of organized atrial activity that occurs with the onset of A Fib.

The second reason that patients with new-onset A Fib are more likely to develop heart failure relates to shortening of the period of ventricular filling. As illustrated on page 17- the period of mechanical ***systole*** (i.e., ventricular contraction) corresponds *approximately* to the period (on an ECG) that begins *just after* the onset of the QRS complex- and continues until the latter portion of the T wave. The period of ***diastole*** (i.e., ventricular *relaxation* and *filling*) begins *after* systole is complete- and continues until the onset of the next QRS complex. Development of *any* tachycardia will *disproportionately* shorten the period of ventricular diastole compared to the period of ventricular systole (which remains relatively constant- *regardless* of the heart rate). As a result, the amount of time available for passive ventricular filling will be significantly curtailed when the ventricular response is rapid- as it most commonly is at the onset of this arrhythmia.

Clinical Notes → Management of A Fib requires a multifaceted approach. This includes use of *"rate-slowing"* drugs (i.e., digoxin, diltiazem, verapamil)- use of other antiarrhythmic agents such as quinidine or procainamide to convert the rhythm to sinus- synchronized cardioversion (for selected patients who fail to respond to medical therapy)- long-term anticoagulation (or at least use of aspirin) to reduce the risk of thromboembolism- and most importantly, a search to identify and correct (if possible) the underlying cause of the A Fib (i.e., heart failure, Acute MI, hyperthyroidism, hyoxemia, etc.).

<u>**Practice**</u>: *Is the rhythm A Fib?*

Both of the rhythms shown below are *irregularly irregular.* However- only *one* of them represents atrial fibrillation. *Which one?* (Explain the rationale for your answer.)

<u>HINT</u>- Do you see P waves in one of these rhythms?

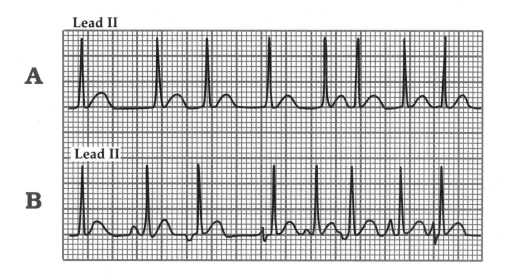

Answer:

Both of the rhythms that appear page 109 are irregularly irregular. There is no atrial activity at all in the top rhythm strip (Example A)- so that this tracing must be the one that represents **atrial fibrillation**. Note that most R-R intervals are *between* 2 large boxes (or even a little less!)- and 3 large boxes- so that the rhythm reflects A Fib with a **rapid** ventricular response. Note also that *no fib waves* are seen in this example- so that the diagnosis of A Fib rests solely on recognition of an *irregularly irregular* rhythm in the *absence* of P waves.

In contrast, P waves *are* present in Example B. Thus despite the fact that this lower rhythm strip on page 109 is also irregularly irregular- this rhythm *can't* be A Fib! Note in particular that the P waves in this example exhibit a striking change in morphology from one P wave to the next- *as well as* a change in the PR interval that precedes each QRS complex. This suggests that P waves in this tracing originate from **M**ultiple different sites in the **A**tria- which, when considered in conjunction with the finding of **T**achycardia (the rate here averages *over* 100 beats/minute)- explains the term **MAT** (**M**ultifocal **A**trial **T**achycardia) that is used to describe this arrhythmia.

> **Clinical Notes** → MAT is a much less common arrhythmia than A Fib. The occurrence of MAT is almost exclusively limited to patients with COPD (chronic obstructive pulmonary disease) or those with severe systemic illness (i.e., sepsis, shock, acid-base or electrolyte abnormalities- or any combination thereof). The importance of recognizing MAT- and distinguishing it from A Fib- *is that treatment of these two conditions is markedly different* ! The treatment of choice for MAT is to identify and correct the underlying/causative disorder. Digoxin should only be used with extreme caution (if at all)- because of the marked predisposition for patients with MAT to develop digitalis toxicity.

Atrial Flutter

Use the **4 *Question Approach*** to interpret the rhythm shown below.

Lead II

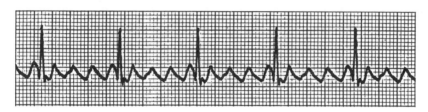

KEY Questions:

1. Is there evidence of *atrial* activity?

2. Are *normal* sinus P waves present?

3. Why is this rhythm *not* atrial fibrillation?

Interpretation:

Applying the **4 Question Approach** to the rhythm that appears on page 111- we note the following:

i) The QRS complex is *narrow* (i.e., *not more* than *half* a large box in duration). This means that the rhythm must be *SUPRAventricular*- and is likely to be one of the entities listed on page 101.

ii) The rhythm is *regular*. The R-R interval is just *over* 4 large boxes in duration- so that the ventricular rate is *about* **70 beats/minute**. Regularity of the ventricular response *rules out* A Fib as a possibility.

iii) & iv) Atrial activity *is* present- but *NOT* in the form of normal sinus P waves. Instead, a *sawtooth* pattern of atrial activity is seen- which defines this rhythm as **Atrial Flutter**.

Clinical Notes → Atrial Flutter is a special type of *supraventricular* rhythm- in which atrial activity almost *magically* occurs at a rate of **300 beats/minute** (usual range = 250-350/minute in the *untreated* patient).

Atrial flutter is an *organized* atrial rhythm- in which there is *rhythmic* (i.e., *regularly* repetitive) flutter activity. Electrocardiographically, this presents as a **sawtooth pattern**- in which each "*tooth*" in the "saw" is occurring at the *magical* rate (i.e., either right at- or very *close to* 300/minute). Note how the rhythm on page 111 displays this *sawtooth* pattern of flutter regularity- with the space between each "tooth" being *approximately* equal to one large box in duration- which corresponds to a rate for the flutter of *about* 300/minute.

In contrast to atrial flutter- **A Fib** is a *chaotic* atrial rhythm in which atrial activity is completely *disorganized*. Like a bowl of jello placed on a shaking table- the fibrillating atria *never* undergo the same movement twice. Electrocardiographically, fibrillating atrial activity is represented by **fib waves** (page 106). Meaningful atrial contraction is impossible.

<u>A Fib</u> and <u>Atrial Flutter</u>

- A *Clinical* Comparison -

There are many similarities in the clinical approach to management of *A Fib* and *Atrial Flutter.* There are also some important differences- most of which can be explained by reflecting on the nature of atrial acitvity in these two conditions.

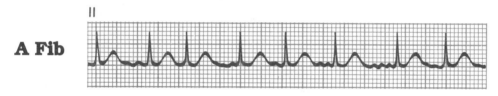

A Fib

Atrial Flutter

<u>Questions:</u>

1. For which rhythm would you expect the risk of thromboembolism to be highest? (i.e., which rhythm disturbance is most likely to predispose to development of clot from *stasis* of blood within the atria?)

2. Which rhythm would you expect to most readily respond to *synchronized* cardioversion?

Answers:

As discussed on page 112- a fundamental difference between *A Fib* and *Atrial Flutter* is that the latter is an *organized* atrial rhythm- and the former is not. Because contractile movements of fibrillating atria are ineffective, cardiac output is reduced (i.e., the "atrial kick" is lost)- and conditions are set up that predispose to *stasis* and clot formation within the atria. This in turn produces a marked propensity toward thromboembolism. Thus, the presence of *chronic* A Fib is the single most important risk factor for development of stroke- which is why long-term **anticoagulation** (or at least treatment with *aspirin*) should be strongly considered in all such patients. In contrast to A Fib- atrial activity with flutter *is* organized- albeit at an exceedingly rapid rate (of close to 300/minute). As a result, patients with atrial flutter are *not* nearly as predisposed to conditions of stasis and clot formation within the atria- and anticoagulation is therefore much less likely to be needed!

It is important to emphasize that in clinical practice, A Fib is a far more commonly occurring arrhythmia than atrial flutter. This is especially true in the elderly- in whom the incidence of A Fib is *at least* 5%. In general, the *identical* drugs are used to treat *both* arrhythmias- including **rate-slowing agents** (i.e., digoxin, verapamil, diltiazem, and/or beta-blockers)- as well as **drugs** used for attempting **to convert the rhythm** to sinus (i.e., quinidine, procainamide, flecainide, amiodarone, and sotalol- *among others*). Unfortunately- despite the use of even high-dose antiarrhythmic therapy- the ventricular response to atrial flutter will often be resistent to medical treatment and remain excessively rapid. In contrast- use of *rate-slowing* drugs is much more likely to be effective in controlling the ventricular response of A Fib.

The opposite response occurs with respect to the use of **synchronized cardioversion**. That is, atrial flutter will typically be very *sensitive* to cardioversion (and will usually respond to low energy attempts with 50 joules or less)- whereas A Fib is much less likely to respond to cardioversion, and often requires higher energies (usually of ≥200 joules) to be successful.

Atrial Flutter

- ECG *Clues* to Diagnosis -

In our experience- ***Atrial Flutter*** is the most frequently *overlooked* cardiac arrhythmia (*by far!*). Simple awareness of the most common atrial and ventricular rates that are likely to be associated with flutter may prove invaluable in facilitating recognition of this arrhythmia.

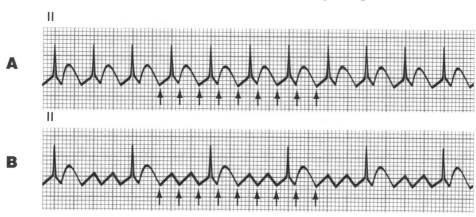

Questions:

1. What is the *atrial* rate of flutter activity for the two example tracings shown above? (<u>HINT</u>- *At what rate are the arrowheads occurring?*)

2. Would you think it desirable for every atrial impulse with flutter to be conducted to the ventricles? If not- *why not*?

Answers:

Flutter activity is occurring at a rate of **300/minute** for both of the rhythms that are shown on the preceding page- as evidenced by the fact that the distance *between* each flutter wave is *exactly* one large box in duration (*See arrowheads in each Figure on page 115*). As emphasized on page 112- this is precisely the rate that is most commonly seen with this arrhythmia.

It is fortunate that *NOT* every atrial impulse with flutter will usually be conducted to the ventricles. If every impulse was conducted- then the ventricular response would *also* be 300 beats/minute- which is far too rapid a response to allow adequate ventricular filling. Instead, a *physiologic* "block" to AV conduction usually occurs- with the result that the most common *ventricular* response (*by far!*) to atrial flutter is with **2:1 AV conduction**. Given the usual atrial flutter rate of *about* **300/minute**- this means that *most* of the time the ventricular rate of a patient with *untreated* atrial flutter will be *very close* to **150 beats/minute** (i.e., ≈300 ÷ 2). This relationship (i.e., of atrial flutter with 2:1 AV conduction) is well illustrated by Example A that appears on page 115. Note in particular that there are 2 flutter waves (*arrowheads*) for every QRS- and that the R-R interval *between* QRS complexes is *exactly* 2 large boxes in duration- which corresponds to the expected ventricular rate of 150 beats/minute.

Next to 2:1 AV conduction, the second most common ventricular response to atrial flutter is with **4:1 AV conduction**. At the usual atrial flutter rate of approximately 300/minute- this typically results in a *ventricular* rate that usually is quite *close to* **75 beats/minute** (i.e., ≈300 ÷ 4)- as shown in Example B on page 115 (as well as for the rhythm on page 111).

Note → It is ever so much *easier* to recognize the typical *sawtooth* pattern of atrial flutter when the ventricular response is *slower* (as it is on page 115 in Example B which manifests 4:1 AV conduction)- than it is when there is 2:1 AV conduction (as in Example A).

Atrial Flutter

- with *Variable* AV Conduction -

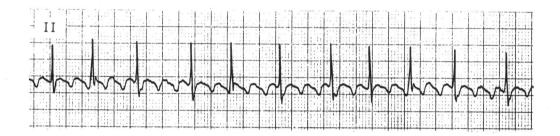

Questions:

1. Despite the fact that the above rhythm is *irregularly* irregular- it is *not* A Fib. *Why not?*

2. How can you tell *at a glance* that the mechanism of this rhythm is definitely *not* sinus?

Answer:

The rhythm that appears on the preceding page is rapid- *irregularly* irregular- and *SUPRAventricular* (since the QRS complex is narrow). However, despite irregularity of the ventricular response- this rhythm is *not* A Fib. The rhythm *can't* be A Fib- because regularly occurring *atrial* activity (in the form of repetitive *negative* deflections) is once again seen *throughout* the rhythm strip. The rate of these negative deflections is *approximately* 300/minute- which once again identifies the rhythm as ***Atrial Flutter-*** in this case with a ***variable*** *ventricular response.*

Ventricular Responses to Atrial Flutter:

- The most common ventricular response (*by far!*) to atrial flutter is with a **2:1 AV conduction ratio**. Given the usual atrial rate (of ≈300/minute for the *untreated* patient with flutter)- this will most commonly result in a *ventricular* response of *close to* **150 beats/minute** (*See page 116*).

- The next most common ventricular response is with a **4:1 AV conduction ratio** (i.e., atrial rate ≈300/minute; ventricular rate ≈75/minute).

- *ODD conduction ratios to atrial flutter* (i.e., with 1:1, 3:1, or 5:1 AV conduction) *are exceedingly uncommon-* if not rare!

- Atrial flutter may occasionally present with a ***variable* AV conduction ratio** (as it does on page 117). Next to 2:1 and 4:1 AV conduction- *variable* AV conduction is probably the third most common ventricular response to atrial flutter.

Note → We know *at a glance* that the rhythm on page 117 *CAN'T* be sinus- *because there is NO upright P wave in standard lead II.*

Atrial Flutter

- Why 12 Leads are Better than One -

The 12-lead ECG shown below was obtained from a patient in atrial flutter. *Does this tracing help to explain why atrial flutter is so frequently overlooked?* (<u>HINT</u>- Look in *all* 12 leads for signs of atrial activity.)

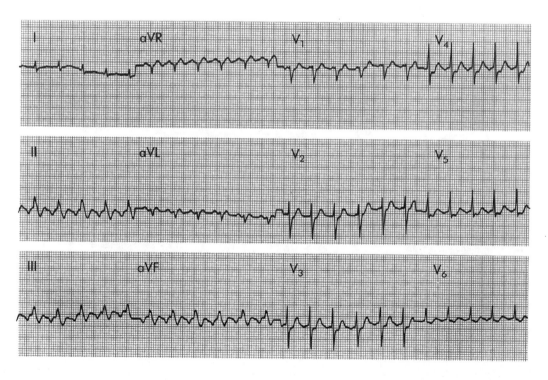

Answers:

The 12-lead ECG that is shown on page 119 can be used to explain why ***Atrial Flutter*** is the most commonly *overlooked* arrhythmia (*by far!*) in clinical practice.

By the *4 Question Approach*, we can say that the rhythm on this tracing is *regular* and *SUPRAventricular* (i.e., the QRS complex is clearly *not more* than half a large box in duration). The heart rate is *very close* to 150 beats/minute (since the R-R interval is *almost exactly* 2 large boxes in duration). Normal sinus P waves are absent (since there is no upright P wave in standard lead II).

For clarification, we show a *simultaneously* recorded rhythm strip (of leads I and II) on this patient. Note the presence of repetitive *negative* deflections that occur at a rate of 300/minute in lead II (*arrows in the Figure below*). Recognition of *regular* atrial activity at a rate that is close to 300/minute *confirms* that this rhythm is atrial flutter. However, there is absolutely *NO indication* of flutter in simultaneously recorded lead I (nor for that matter, on many of the *other* leads on the 12-lead ECG that is shown on page 119).

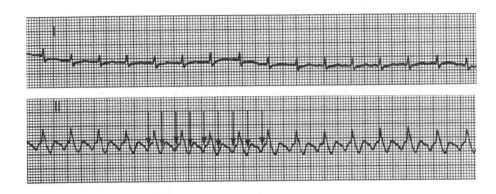

> **Pearl** → The *KEY* to *not* missing the diagnosis of ***Atrial Flutter-*** is to *ALWAYS suspect* this rhythm- *WHENEVER* there is a *regular* SVT (supraventricular tachycardia) at a rate of *about* 150 beats/minute- especially when the nature of atrial activity is uncertain.

Practice: *What is the rhythm?*

Use the **4 *Question* Approach** to interpret the rhythm shown below.

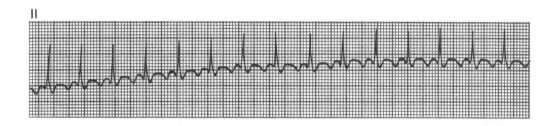

HINT- Given the *regularity* of this rhythm and the *rate* of the ventricular response- *what diagnosis should you suspect ????*

Interpretation:

Applying the **4 *Question Approach*** to the rhythm that appears on page 121- we note the following:

    i) The QRS complex is *narrow* (i.e., *not more* than *half* a large box in duration). This means that the rhythm must be *SUPRAventricular*- and is likely to be one of the entities listed on page 101.

    ii) The rhythm is *regular.* This *rules out* A Fib as a possibility. The R-R interval of this rhythm is almost exactly 2 large boxes in duration- which means that the ventricular rate is *very close* to **150 beats/minute**.

    iii) Atrial activity *is* present- but *NOT* in the form of normal sinus P waves. If the upright deflection preceding each QRS complex was construed as the P wave- the PR interval would be *too short* to be conducted by the normal pathway. If on the other hand the negative deflection preceding each QRS was the P wave- the mechanism of the rhythm still *could not* be sinus because a normal sinus P wave should be *upright* in lead II.

> **<u>Comment</u>** → The presence of a *regular* SVT at a rate of *about* 150 beats/minute- in the *absence* of normal sinus P waves- *should strongly suggest the diagnosis of **Atrial Flutter**.* Although admittedly subtle- flutter waves *are* present in the rhythm that is seen on preceding page (*arrows below*)- emphasizing again the importance of maintaining a high index of suspicion for the diagnosis of flutter- *whenever* there is a *regular* SVT at a rate of *about* 150 beats/minute- in the *absence* of normal atrial activity.

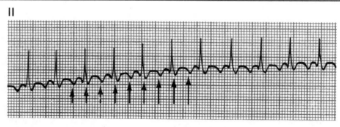

Atrial Flutter

- *Thought-Provoking Questions* -

As a final exercise for understanding the relationship between AV conduction and atrial flutter- consider the *thought-provoking* questions that we pose below. (Feel free to refer to pages 111-122 in formulating your answers.)

Questions:

1. If the atrial rate of a patient in flutter was **280/minute-** what would you expect as the *most likely* ventricular response? as the *next most likely* ventricular response?

2. Imagine instead that the atrial rate was **320/minute.** What rate(s) might you now expect for the ventricular response?

3. Keeping in mind the *usual range* for the atrial rate of an adult patient in flutter (i.e., 250-350/minute)- as well as the most common AV conduction ratios for flutter- *Why should it be so unusual for an UNTREATED adult with a regular ventricular rate of **100 beats/minute** to be in atrial flutter?* for an adult with a regular ventricular rate of **200 beats/ minute** to be in flutter?

Answers:

1. As emphasized earlier- the most common ventricular response to atrial flutter (*by far!*) is with 2:1 AV conduction. This means that if the atrial rate was **280** beats/minute- the ventricular rate is most likely to be **140 beats/minute** (i.e., 280 ÷ 2). The next most common ventricular response to atrial flutter is with 4:1 AV conduction- which should result in a ventricular rate of **70 beats/minute** at a flutter rate of 280 (i.e., 280 ÷ 4).

2. If instead of 280/minute, the atrial rate of a patient in flutter was **320** beats/minute- then a 2:1 AV conduction ratio should result in a ventricular rate of **160 beats/minute** (320 ÷2)- and a 4:1 AV conduction ratio should result in a ventricular rate of **80 beats/minute** (320 ÷ 4).

3. It is highly *unlikely* for an **untreated adult** with a *regular* ventricular response of 100 beats/minute to be in atrial flutter. This is because if atrial flutter was present with 2:1 AV conduction *and* a ventricular rate of 100 beats/minute- the atrial rate would have to be 200/minute (i.e., 100 X 2)- *which is a rate that falls well below the usual range for flutter activity.* For similar reasons, it is equally unlikely for an *untreated* adult with a regular ventricular rate of 200 beats/minute to be in atrial flutter- because this rate is *too slow* for atrial flutter with 1:1 AV conduction- and *too fast* for flutter with 2:1 AV conduction.

Note → There are 2 exceptions to the general rules we cite for the usual atrial range for flutter (i.e., of *between* 250-350/minute):

- **Children**- in whom much *faster* atrial rates (of 400/minute- *or more!*) may be seen. (Fortunately, atrial flutter in children is *rare* !)
- **Treated patients**- in whom use of certain *antiarrhythmic* drugs (i.e., quinidine, procainamide, verapamil, diltiazem- *and others*) may significantly *slow* the *atrial* rate (often to the range of 200-250/minute).

The <u>Regular SVT</u>

- *Differential Diagnosis* -

A common diagnostic problem is to determine the cause of a **Regular NARROW-Complex** (and therefore *SUPRAventricular*) **Tachycardia**- such as the rhythm shown below. There are 3 principal entities to consider:

The Most Common Causes of a Regular SVT :
1. Sinus Tachycardia
2. Atrial Flutter
3. PSVT

Lead II

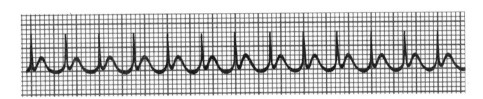

<u>Question:</u>

1. Which of the entities in the above list is the most likely cause of the SVT shown here?

> <u>HINT</u>- Use the **4 Question Approach** to interpret the rhythm- being sure to determine the *heart rate* before answering the Question. (Feel free to refer to pages 97-98 and 123-124 in formulating your answer.)

Section 1C- *SUPRAVentricular* Rhythms

Interpretation:

Applying the **4 *Question Approach*** to the rhythm that appears page 125- we note the following:

i) The QRS complex is *narrow* (i.e., clearly *not more* than *half* a large box in duration)- which means that the rhythm must be *SUPRAventricular.*

ii) The rhythm is *regular.* This *rules out* A Fib as a possibility. The rate is obviously fast- and can best be calculated using the **Every-OTHER-Beat Method** (described on pages 55-58). The method determines the R-R interval of every *other* beat (i.e., *half* the rate)- and then *doubles* this number. Using the first QRS complex in the rhythm strip as our starting point (since this complex *begins* on a *heavy* line)- it can be seen that the R-R interval of every *other* beat (i.e., the R-R interval of *half* the rate) is 3 large boxes in duration. This means that *half* the rate is 100 beats/minute- and that the *actual* rate must therefore be **200 beats/minute**.

iii) & iv) There are no P waves (or other signs of atrial activity).

> **Comment** → The rhythm that appears on page 125 is a *Regular SVT* at a rate of 200 beats/minute- *without* any evidence of atrial activity. Regarding the **Most Common Causes of a Regular SVT** :
>
> 1. *Sinus Tachycardia*- is unlikely given the absence of atrial activity and the rapidity of the rate (i.e., sinus tachycardia *rarely* exceeds 150-160 beats/minute in a non-exercising adult- *See pages 97-98*).
> 2. *Atrial Flutter*- is equally unlikely (assuming the patient is *not* on anti-arrhythmic medication)- since a ventricular rate of 200 beats/minute would seem to be *too slow* for atrial flutter with 1:1 AV conduction- and *too fast* for atrial flutter with 2:1 AV conduction (*See pages 123-124*).
> 3. **PSVT**- must therefore be the diagnosis- by the process of elimination (*See page 127*).

<u>PSVT</u>

(*Paroxysmal SupraVentricular Tachycardia*)

PSVT is a *reentry* tachycardia- in which the electrical impulse gets caught in a cycle that *continuously* circulates around (or within) the AV node- *as suggested by the Figure below*. With *each* revolution, the circulating electrical impulse gives off a branch that is conducted to the ventricles (to produce a QRS complex)- and then *"reenters"* the cycle as it reembarks on another revolution around the AV node.

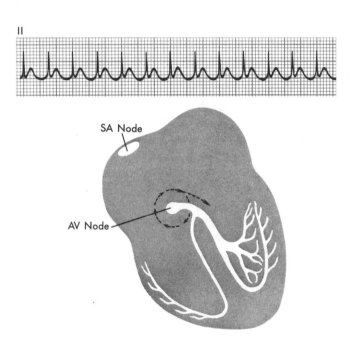

Regarding the Rhythm known as PSVT:

ECG Recognition → Regular supraventricular tachycardia at a rate of *between* 150 to 240 beats/minute- usually *without* obvious sign of atrial activity. On occasion, there may be subtle notching (or a small negative deflection) that deforms the terminal portion of the QRS complex (representing *retrograde* atrial activity)- but most of the time the ECG picture will be similar to that seen on the preceding page (as well as on page 125).

Mechanism → PSVT involves the phenomenon of *AV nodal reentry.* As *schematically* depicted on page 127- the electrical impulse gets caught up in a cycle that *continually* circulates around (or within) the AV node- producing a tachycardia that persists *until* the AV nodal reentry cycle is somehow *interrupted* (i.e., by drugs, vagal maneuvers, or spontaneously).

Terminology → In the past, it was common to refer to the rhythm shown on page 127 as either **PAT** or **PJT** (i.e., *Paroxysmal Atrial* or *Junctional Tachycardia*). This older terminology is no longer recommended because it implies more than we actually know about the etiology of the arrhythmia (since there is really *no way* to tell from just looking at the ECG rhythm whether the arrhythmia originates in the atria or the AV node- or from *neither* site).

In recent years *P*SVT has become the term most commonly used to describe this arrhythmia- in which the **"P"** of the name serves to remind the clinician of how sudden (i.e., *"Paroxysmal"*) the onset of PSVT typically is. Even more recently, a *new* name has been adopted- which is ***AVNRT*** (***AV Nodal Reentry Tachycardia***). Technically, *AVNRT* would seem to be an even *better* term than PSVT- because it emphasizes how the mechanism of the *Tachycardia* almost always involves *Reentry* within (or into) the *AV Node.* Nevertheless, for the purpose of *consistency* with AHA Guidelines- *we elect to refer to this rhythm as* **PSVT** *throughout this book (as well as in our other ACLS materials).*

Terminology- "<u>**SVT**</u>"

(= <u>S</u>upra<u>V</u>entricular <u>T</u>achycardia)

As already emphasized (on pages 80 and 101)- **SUPRAventricular rhythms** are those in which the electrical impluse originates *at* or *above* the AV node (i.e., at or above the *double dotted line* in the Figure below).

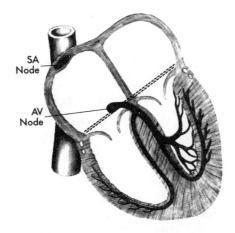

SA
Node

AV
Node

<u>Question:</u>

1. Keeping in mind the above definition for a *SUPRAventricular* rhythm- *how would you define the term* <u>S</u>upra<u>V</u>entricular <u>T</u>achycardia (i.e., "**SVT**")?

<u>HINT</u>- Remember that a *"tachycardia"* is a rhythm with a heart rate of 100 beats/minute or more.

Answers:

The term **<u>SVT</u>** (= **S**upra**V**entricular **T**achycardia) can be viewed as a "generic" one that encompasses *ALL* tachyarrhythmias in which heart rate is ≥**100/minute**- and the impulse *originates* **at** or **above** the AV Node. Unless aberrant conduction or preexisting bundle branch block is present- the QRS complex should be *NARROW* when the rhythm is *SUPRAventricular* (*pages 79-80*).

Entities included within the broad definition of " **<u>SVT</u>** " are:

- ***Sinus Tachycardia***
    - ***Junctional Tachycardia***
      - ***Atrial Fibrillation***
        - ***Atrial Flutter***
          - ***Multifocal Atrial Tachycardia (MAT)***
            - ***Ectopic Atrial Tachycardia***
              - ***PSVT (*or* AVNRT)***

> **<u>Note</u>** → In the past the *generic* term **"SVT"** was used synonymously with PAT, PJT, or PSVT. This practice is potentially misleading because *supraventricular* arrhythmias such as sinus tachycardia constitute a form of SVT that is very *different* from atrial or junctional tachycardia- and from PSVT. We therefore favor reserving use of the term "SVT" as a *general* descriptor for *NARROW-complex* tachycardias of *uncertain* etiology- and for specifying the *type* of SVT as soon as we know the diagnosis (i.e., using *PSVT* to describe the rhythms that appears on the front of pages 125 and 127).

PSVT

- *Clinical Significance* -

As implied by its name, **P**SVT typically has a *sudden* onset (i.e., it is *"Paroxysmal"*). The tachycardia may either be *short-lived-* or it may last for *hours* (or even for *days* !)- until the reentry cycle terminates *spontaneously-* or is interrupted by treatment.

Clinically, PSVT is probably the most common *sustained* tachyarrhythmia to occur in otherwise healthy young adults. It may also be seen in older individuals who have underlying heart disease.

Lead II

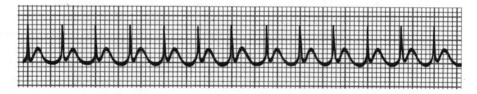

Question:

1. What symptoms would you most commonly expect to see in patients with PSVT?

2. How would you imagine the rhythm is best treated?

> HINT- Remember that the *mechanism* of the rhythm almost always involves *reentry* into (or within) the AV node (*See pages 127-128*).

Answers:

The symptom most commonly seen in patients with PSVT is a sensation of *palpitations.* Since this feeling of "heart racing" may be extremely disturbing to the patient, the tachycardia is often associated with acute anxiety. Other common symptoms include chest discomfort and shortness of breath.

Hemodynamically, most patients tolerate PSVT surprisingly well- even when the rate is rapid (*between* 200-240 beats/minute) and the rhythm long lasting. On occasion, however- *hypotension* and/or *heart failure* may develop- especially in older patients (or in very young children)- and especially when the rate of PSVT is more rapid- the rhythm is sustained- and/or underlying heart disease is present.

Clinically, many treatment options are available for PSVT. The modality (or modalities) selected will usually depend on the patient's clinical condition and hemodynamic status- as well as personal preference of the treating clinician. Application of a *vagal maneuver* is generally tried first (*See pages 133-138*). If this is not effective and the patient is tolerating the arrhythmia- an *antiarrhythmic* agent (i.e., adenosine, verapamil, diltiazem, or a ß-blocker) is usually tried next. *Antianxiety* medication (i.e., use of a rapidly acting *benzodiazepine*) may be helpful in treatment from *both* a symptomatic standpoint (to reduce anxiety and attenuate the sensation of palpitations)- as well as from a physiologic standpoint (to reduce sympathetic tone and hopefully alter conduction properties within the reentry circuit responsible for sustaining the arrhythmia). *Synchronized cardioversion* is usually reserved for patients who become hemodynamically unstable from PSVT- and/or when other measures fail.

KEY → The common denominator for *all* modalities used in the treatment of PSVT (i.e., vagal maneuvers- anxiolytics- antiarrhythmic agents- and/or cardioversion) is the potential to alter conduction properties *within* the reentry circuit responsible for propagation of the arrhythmia. Even *momentary* delay (as produced by a vagal maneuver) may be enough to *interrupt* the circuit- and therefore terminate the arrhythmia.

Diagnostic Dilemmas

- When the cause of SVT is NOT readily apparent -

Examine again the tracing below- which was initially shown on page 121. Work through the *Differential Diagnosis* we presented on page 125 for the *Most Common Causes of a* **Regular SVT**.

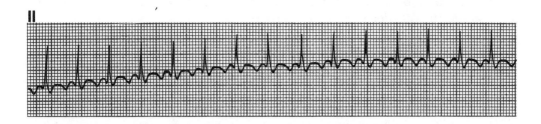

Question:

1. Is there evidence of *atrial* activity? of *normal* atrial activity?

2. What might be done to make atrial activity more apparent?

Answers:

As discussed on page 122, the rhythm that appears on pages 121 and 133 is a *regular SVT* at a rate of about 150 beats/minute. Atrial activity *is* seen- but *not* in the form of normal sinus P waves (i.e., the P wave is *not* upright in this standard lead II). Instead, *negative* deflections that most likely represent *flutter* activity are seen in this lead. As emphasized on pages 120 and 122- the *KEY* to recognizing **Atrial Flutter** is to *ALWAYS* maintain a high index of suspicion for this diagnosis- *WHENEVER* you encounter a *regular* SVT at a rate that is *almost* 150 beats/minute- especially when normal sinus P waves are absent.

Two interventions may be considered in an effort to render atrial activity more apparent- and hopefully *solidify* the diagnosis of *atrial flutter* :

1. Viewing the tracing in *additional* leads (and/or obtaining a 12-lead ECG)- since flutter activity will often be seen better in some leads than in others (*See page 119*).

2. Applying a **VAGAL Maneuver**- in an attempt to *slow* the ventricular response *momentarily*. In so doing, one hopes to uncover *telltale* atrial activity that had previously been hidden within the tachycardia. Application of **Carotid Sinus Massage** (**CSM**- *in the Figure below*) to the rhythm that appears on the pre-ceeding page does just that- *reducing* the ratio of AV conduction (from 2:1 to 4:1)- and allowing *confirmation* of underlying flutter activity at a rate of 300/minute (*arrows in the Figure below*).

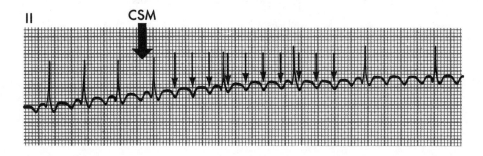

VAGAL MANEUVERS:

CSM- *Mechanism of Action*
- Technique
- Adverse Effects

Note → Although **C**arotid **S**inus **M**assage **(CSM)** is probably the most commonly employed vagal maneuver- there are *many* others. These include:

1. Activation of the gag reflex
2. Performance of *Valsalva*
3. Breath-holding
4. Facial submersion in ice
5. Eyeball pressure (*which is no longer recommended*)
6. Squatting
7. Digital rectal massage

All vagal maneuvers share a common mechanism of action and exert similar antiarrhythmic effects.

P.S. → Some clinicians use administration of **Adenosine** diagnostically as a *"chemical form"* of vagal maneuver. The marked *rate-slowing* effect of this drug may allow detection of atrial activity that had previously been hidden *within* the tachycardia. The extremely short duration of action of this drug (*less* than 10 seconds!)- makes it unlikely that adverse effects will occur.

CSM *(Carotid Sinus Massage):*

Mechanism of Action → Production of a *transient* increase in parasympathetic tone that results in momentary *slowing* of conduction through supraventricular and AV nodal tissues- *while* the maneuver is being applied.

Technique for CSM → Under *constant* ECG monitoring- turn the patient's head to the *left* and gently but *firmly* massage the area of the *RIGHT* carotid bifurcation (near the angle of the jaw!) for 3-5 seconds at a time. After several attempts on the right carotid, the other side may be tried. *NEVER do both sides at once* !

- The *RIGHT* carotid is believed to exert a greater influence on the SA node; the *LEFT* on the AV node.

- Be sure to apply *enough* pressure- in the *correct* location (i.e., *high* in the neck near the *angle* of the jaw!)- and for *no more than* 5 seconds at a time! You may want to warn the patient that the procedure is likely to be *uncomfortable*- and may *even* hurt a little. (The amount of pressure that should be applied is comparable to that needed to squeeze and *indent* a tennis ball.)

Adverse Effects → *CSM is NOT completely benign.* The procedure has been associated with syncope, stroke, sinus arrest, AV block, asystole, and ventricular arrhythmias in patients with digitalis toxicity.

- Be sure to listen to the neck *BEFORE* applying CSM. *Do NOT do the procedure if a carotid bruit is heard* (because you *could* dislodge a plaque and cause a stroke).

VAGAL MANEUVERS:

- *Effect of CSM on various tachyarrhythmias*

Clinical Notes → It should be emphasized that application of a vagal maneuver may not only be a *diagnostic* procedure- but it may also be *therapeutic* ! Thus, the *transient* slowing of conduction that the maneuver produces may either *interrupt* a reentry pathway that involves the AV node (as occurs with *abrupt* termination of PSVT)- or it may *reduce* temporarily the number of impulses able to pass through to the ventricles. Reducing the ventricular rate in this manner may *unmask* previously hidden atrial activity- and in so doing reveal the mechanism of the underlying rhythm (as is seen on page 134).

Effect of CSM (and other Vagal Maneuvers) on Various Tachyarrhythmias

<u>*Tachyarrhythmia*</u>	<u>*Response to CSM*</u>
▪ **Sinus Tachycardia**	- *Gradual slowing* of the sinus tachycardia during CSM- with resumption of the tachycardia *after* the maneuver.
▪ **PSVT**	- *Abrupt termination* of the tachy-arrhythmia (with conversion to sinus rhythm)- <u>OR</u> . . . . *NO response at all to CSM.*
▪ **Atrial Flutter or Fibrillation**	- Increased degree of AV block with *transient* slowing of the ventri-cular rate- that will hopefully allow diagnosis of the arrhythmia by *uncovering* (or clarifying the nature of) previously hidden atrial activity.
▪ **VT**	- *NO response to CSM*

Practice: *What is the rhythm?*

Use the **4 Question Approach** to interpret the rhythm shown below. (<u>HINT</u>- Be sure to use **calipers** for assessing the *regularity* of this rhythm.)

Lead II

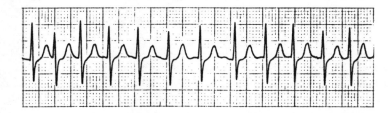

Question → What effect would you expect a *vagal maneuver* to have on this rhythm? (Feel free to refer to the table on page 138 in formulating your answer.)

Interpretation:

Applying the **4 *Question Approach*** to the rhythm that appears on page 139- we note the following:

i) The QRS complex is *narrow* (i.e., clearly *not more* than *half* a large box in duration)- which means that the rhythm must be *SUPRAventricular.*

ii) On initial inspection, it may *appear* that this rhythm is regular. *It is not*! Careful measurement *with* **calipers** reveals that the R-R interval *continually* changes from one beat to the next (i.e., the rhythm is *irregularly* irregular).

iii) & iv) There are no P waves (or other signs of atrial activity).

Comment → The presence of an *irregularly* irregular rhythm in the *absence* of atrial activity- defines this rhythm to be **Atrial Fibrillation**- in this case with a **rapid ventricular response**. Fib waves are *not* seen on this tracing (*See pages 105-106*).

　　The clinical point to emphasize is that A Fib may sometimes *simulate* PSVT when the ventricular response is rapid (as it is for the rhythm that appears on page 139). This may affect therapeutic decision-making because treatment of these 2 conditions will often be quite different. For example, *adenosine* is the drug of choice for PSVT- but it is ineffective for A Fib; *digoxin* is still preferred by many for treatment of A Fib- but its onset of action is too delayed for optimal use with PSVT.

　　Application of a *vagal maneuver* to the rhythm that appears on page 139 might help to resolve any areas of diagnostic uncertainty. As indicated on page 138- application of a vagal manevuer to a patient in A Fib would be expected to transiently *decrease* the number of impulses transmitted to the ventricles. Although this *won't* convert A Fib to sinus rhythm- it might *confirm* the diagnosis (if confirmation was needed) by clarifying the nature of atrial activity.

<u>Practice</u>: *What is the Rhythm?*

The rhythm shown below is *regular* and clearly *SUPRAventricular* (since the QRS complex is *not more* than half a large box in duration). Which of the entities listed on page 101 is this rhythm most likely to be?

Lead II

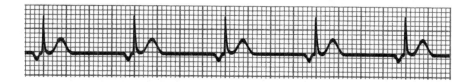

<u>Questions:</u>

1. Is there evidence of *atrial* activity? of *normal* atrial activity?

2. From where in the heart would you expect this rhythm to originate?

Answer:

As noted, the rhythm that appears on the preceeding page is *regular* and *SUPRAventricular* (since the QRS complex is clearly *not more* than half a large box in duration). The heart rate is **75 beats/minute**. P waves *are* present- but they are **negative** in this standard lead II. This means that the rhythm can *not* be sinus. Instead, the rhythm originates from the AV node. Note from the Figure below how the *direction* of atrial depolarization is *retrograde* when the electrical impulse originates from the AV node- which is why the P wave appears as a *negative* deflection in standard lead II with an **AV nodal (junctional) rhythm**.

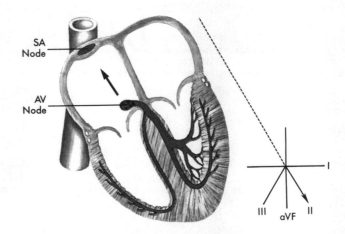

> **Note** → We have *already* seen the rhythm that appears on page 141 (i.e., on page 77). As emphasized on that page- and on pages 74-76- the importance of finding a *negative* P wave in standard lead II is that this essentially *rules out* a sinus mechanism for the rhythm (assuming of course, that the patient does *not* have dextrocardia or lead misplacement).

Junctional (AV Nodal) Rhythm

- P wave Polarity -

As noted on page 142- the P wave in standard lead II is *negative* with an AV nodal (junctional) rhythm. This will produce one of 3 possible patterns of P wave polarity (labeled **B**, **C**, and **D** in the *laddergram* below):

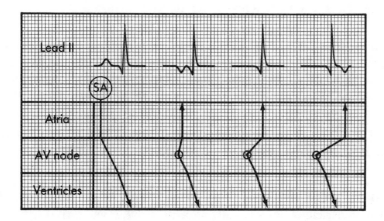

> **Note** → With a normal sinus rhythm (NSR)- the P wave will be *upright* in standard lead II (**Complex A** above). This is because of the *forward* direction of atrial depolarization (which *begins* in the SA node). In contrast, with AV nodal rhythms- the P wave in lead II will be *negative* (i.e., *retrograde*) and appear *before* the QRS (**Complex B**)- be *hidden* by the QRS (**Complex C**)- or appear *after* the QRS (**Complex D**).

P Wave Polarity with Junctional Rhythms

The Figure that appears on page 143 is a **laddergram.** Use of this schematic teaching modality is an optimal way to illustrate the *sequence* of cardiac conduction and the mechanism of various arrhythmias. In this particular example, the laddergram allows us to compare P wave morphology in lead II during NSR- with the patterns that may be seen with an AV nodal (junctional) rhythm.

- **Complex A**- which is the pattern for **NSR**- in which the impulse begins in the SA node and *sequentially* travels through the atria (upper tier in the laddergram), AV node (middle tier), and the ventricles (lower tier).

> In contrast to what happens with NSR- with **junctional rhythms** the electrical impulse originates within the *middle* (AV nodal) tier. From the AV node, the impulse then travels backward (*retrograde*) to depolarize the atria- *as well as* forward (*antegrade*) to depolarize the ventricles. One of 3 possible patterns may be seen:

- **Complex B**- in which retrograde atrial conduction is *faster* than antegrade conduction to the ventricles. This results in a negative P wave (with a short PR interval) that appears *before* the QRS complex in lead II.

- **Complex D**- in which retrograde atrial conduction is *slower* than antegrade conduction to the ventricles. This results in a negative P wave that appears *after* the QRS complex in lead II.

- **Complex C**- in which retrograde atrial conduction takes approximately the *same amount* of time as antegrade conduction to the ventricles. As a result, atrial activity will be hidden *within* the QRS complex- and no P wave at all will be seen in lead II. Clinically, this pattern is the one that occurs most commonly in practice.

<u>Junctional Rhythms</u>

- ECG Recognition (rate/P waves) -

Examine the 3 examples of ***junctional rhythm*** that are shown below. Keeping in mind the 3 possible patterns of P wave polarity (presented on page 143)- comment on the presence (and nature) of atrial activity in each of these examples.

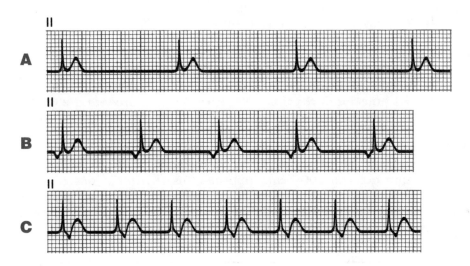

<u>**Additional Question**</u> → Keeping in mind that the usual (i.e., "normal") rate of an AV nodal (junctional) rhythm in an *adult* is *between* **40-60 beats/minute**- *Is the rate for each of the above examples comparable to what you would expect?*

Answer:

We note several similarities between the 3 examples of ***junctional rhythm*** that appear on the preceeding page. Specifically- each rhythm is *regular*- and the QRS complex is uniformly *narrow*. Distinction between these rhythms is a function of the difference in heart rate and the nature of atrial activity.

- **Example A**- The R-R interval is 6 large boxes in duration- which corresponds to a heart rate of **50 beats/minute**. This rate falls *within* the usual range for an **AV nodal *escape* rhythm** in adults (i.e., *between* 40-60 beats/minute). No P waves at all are seen on this tracing- so that this pattern corresponds to **Complex C** (that appeared on page 143).

- **Example B**- The R-R interval is 4 large boxes in duration- which corresponds to a heart rate of **75 beats/minute**. Since this rate clearly *exceeds* the usual rate associated with an AV nodal escape pacemaker- this rhythm is described as an **accelerated junctional rhythm**. Negative P waves *precede* the QRS- so that this pattern corresponds to **Complex B** (that appeared on page 143).

- **Example C**- The R-R interval is *less* than 3 large boxes in duration- which corresponds to a heart rate of *about* **110 beats/minute**. Since the rate of this junctional rhythm exceeds 100 beats/minute- this rhythm is described as **junctional *tachycardia***. Atrial activity *is* present- in the form of negative P waves that follow *just after* the QRS- so that this pattern corresponds to **Complex D** (that appeared on page 143).

> **Note** → Technically speaking it may *not* be possible to distinguish between a junctional rhythm that produces negative P waves that precede the QRS complex (as seen in the middle tracing page 145)- and a *low atrial rhythm* in which the electrical impulse originates from a point that is anatomically close to the AV node. Fortunately this distinction is largely academic- since the clinical significance of a low atrial rhythm is virtually *identical* to that of a junctional rhythm.

Junctional Rhythms

- Types and Clinical Significance -

Junctional rhythms are classified into one of 3 types on the basis of the *rate* of the rhythm:

- **AV Nodal *Escape* Rhythm**- when the rate is *between* 40-60 beats/minute which is the usual rate of an AV nodal "escape" pacemaker. This corresponds to *Example A* on page 145.

- **Accelerated Junctional Rhythm**- when the rate is *between* 61-99 beats/ minute. This corresponds to *Example B* on page 145.

- **Junctional *Tachycardia*-** when the rate is *at least* 100 beats/minute. This corresponds to *Example C* on page 145.

Clinical Notes → It should be apparent that for practical purposes the terms ***AV nodal* rhythm** and ***junctional* rhythm** are synonyms. We therefore use these terms interchangeably throughout this book.

It should be emphasized that the difference between an "accelerated" junctional rhythm and junctional "tachycardia" is largely semantic and a function of heart rate. Technically- an *accelerated* junctional rhythm *becomes* junctional "tachycardia" once the heart rate attains 100 beats/minute or more. Clinically- the significance of these two rhythms is virtually identical.

Clinical Significance of the Junctional Rhythms

The significance of the various junctional rhythms depends most on the clinical setting in which they occur. Development of an **AV nodal *escape* rhythm** with an *appropriate* escape rate (i.e., a *nonaccelerated* junctional rate of between 40-60 beats/minute) should therefore be interpreted as a *normal* finding when it occurs in otherwise healthy young adults. This is especially true when this rhythm occurs in the setting of certain predisposing conditions (i.e., relaxation states, at the onset of sleep or induction of anesthesia, and with intense physical conditioning). Each of these conditions is commonly associated with intermittent reduction in the rate of the normal sinus pacemaker. ***Default*** of the pacemaking function from the SA node to a *standby* junctional pacemaker having a set point at a slightly higher rate is perfectly *appropriate* in such clinical settings- and should *not* be cause for alarm. If anything- development of an AV nodal rhythm at an appropriate "escape" rate (of say, 50 beats/minute)- would seem *preferable* to marked "physiologic" sinus bradycardia at a much slower rate (i.e., of *less* than 40 beats/minute).

On the other hand- abrupt development of the same AV nodal escape rhythm in an elderly patient in response to a syncopal episode (that had been precipitated by marked sinus bradycardia) should prompt a very different conclusion. In this situation- the marked sinus bradycardia and *resultant* AV nodal escape rhythm are likely to be *pathologic* manifestations of *sick sinus syndrome* in this symptomatic patient who will almost certainly need a permanent pacemaker.

In contrast to situations in which *physiologic* sinus node slowing occurs (with resultant ***default*** of the pacemaking function to a standby junctional pacemaker)- *takeover* (i.e, ***usurpation***) of the rhythm by *acceleration* of the AV nodal rhythm (i.e., to a rate of *more* than 60 beats/minute) is almost always pathologic. Clinically, the three conditions most likely to cause an ***accelerated* junctional rhythm** and/or **junctional *tachycardia*** are digitalis toxicity, acute inferior infarction, and the post-operative state.

> **Note** → Although many patients maintain normal hemodynamic function with junctional rhythm- hypotension may occur as a result of the fact that the "atrial kick" is lost.

Practice: *What is the Rhythm?*

Use the **4 Question Approach** to interpret the rhythm shown below.

Lead II

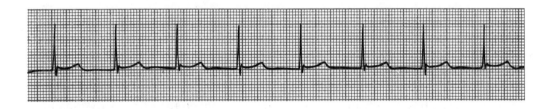

Questions:

    1. Would application of a vagal maneuver be helpful in the diagnostic process?

    2. Is the heart rate for the above tracing what you would normally expect for this type of rhythm?

Interpretation:

Applying the **4 Question Approach** to the rhythm that appears on page 149- we note the following:

i) The QRS complex is *narrow* (i.e., clearly *not more* than *half* a large box in duration)- which means that the rhythm must be *SUPRAventricular.*

ii) The rhythm is *regular.* The R-R interval is just *over* 4 large boxes in duration- which corresponds to a rate of *about* **72 beats/minute**.

iii) & iv) There are no P waves (or other signs of atrial activity).

Comment → The presence of a *regular* supraventricular rhythm *without* evidence of atrial activity defines this as a junctional rhythm. Since the heart rate is *greater* than the 40-60 beat/minute range usually anticipated for an AV nodal *escape* rhythm- this rhythm qualifies as an **accelerated junctional rhythm**.

Use of a vagal maneuver is *not* needed (and would *not* be helpful) in the diagnostic process- because the rate of this rhythm is *not* rapid.   Application of a vagal maneuver is primarily used when the rate of a supraventricular rhythm is fast (i.e., usually well *over* 120 beats/minute)- in the hope of slowing the ventricular response enough to *uncover* underlying atrial activity (*See pages 137-138*).   It should be clear in this case *without* the need for additional slowing that atrial activity is definitely absent.

Note → The usual range cited for the expected rate of an AV nodal escape rhythm in **adults** is between 40-60 beats/minute.   The range is different for **children**- in whom a rate range of between 50-80 beats/minute is the norm.   Thus, an AV nodal rhythm in a child should *not* be considered "accelerated" unless the rate *exceeds* 80 beats/minute.

Section 1D- *Premature Beats/VT*

Early and *Late* Beats

- ECG Recognition -

In *Section 1B* we emphasized the importance of determining the *overall* pattern of rhythm regularity for every arrhythmia you encounter. In addition to this overall pattern- unexpectedly *EARLY* or *LATE* beats may occur that alter the underlying pattern of the general rhythm. Reexamine this concept in the two schematic tracings shown below.

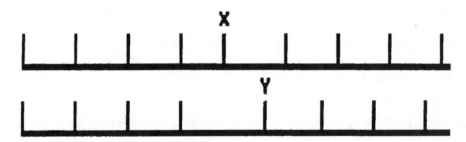

Question:

1. Do the complexes labeled " **X** " and " **Y** " in the above examples interrupt the *underlying* pattern of rhythm regularity by occurring *early* or *late* ?

HINT- Feel free to refer back to pages 67-68 in formulating your answer.

Answer:

As discussed on pages 63-72- an essential facet of arrhythmia interpretation is to determine the *underlying* pattern of regularity for the rhythm being analyzed. When the underlying rhythm is regular (or at least *fairly* regular)- it will usually be easy to recognize *EARLY*-occurring (i.e., **premature**) and *LATE*-occurring (i.e., **escape**) beats.

Both of the examples that appear on page 151 exhibit a pattern of underlying *regularity*-with the exception of the beats labeled "X" and "Y" (and the interval that immediately follows these complexes). The complex labeled " **X** " interrupts the pattern by occurring *early*. In contrast- the complex labeled " **Y** " interrupts the pattern by occuring *late.*

- Clinical examples of **EARLY**-*occurring* beats include PACs, PJCs, and PVCs (i.e., *premature* atrial, junctional, and ventricular contractions). These beats are discussed on pages 155, 157 and 161.

- **LATE**-*occurring* beats are perhaps best thought of as *protective*- in that they most often reflect *"escape"* activity arising from a lower pacemaker (with the specific goal of preventing excessive bradycardia). The concept of escape beats (and escape rhythms) is discussed more fully in <u>Section 1E</u> (*that begins on page 191).*

<u>Pearl</u> → A *KEY* concept to master in arrhythmia interpretation relates to the process of what to do when the "theme" of a *portion* of an arrhythmia differs from the picture present on the rest of the rhythm strip. *Judgement is needed to determine the* **true underlying pattern.** For example- in the two schematic tracings that appear on page 151- recognition that the *underlying* pattern of each rhythm is regular is essential before being able to proceed in determining whether beats "X" and "Y" are early or late.

> In general- when a rhythm strip contains information that is *easy* to evaluate- *as well as* information that is more difficult to evaluate- we suggest you begin **first with that part of the tracing that is *easiest* to interpret.**

Types of *Premature* Beats

Premature beats are beats that interrupt the underlying rhythm by occurring *earlier* than expected. As alluded to on pages 151-152- they are of 3 basic types:

- *PACs* (*Premature Atrial Contractions*)

- *PJCs* (*Premature Junctional Contractions*)

- *PVCs* (*Premature Ventricular Contractions*)

Questions:

1. Which of the types of premature beats will be preceded by a *premature* (i.e., *early* occurring) P wave? *How should these premature P waves look?*

2. How should the QRS complex look for each of the types of premature beats?

HINT- Feel free to refer back to pages 15-16 in formulating your answer.

Answer:

PACs are *early* occurring beats that arise from somewhere in the atria *other than* the SA node. As a result, they will be *preceded* by a premature P wave that usually looks quite different from the normal sinus P wave (since by definition, a PAC arises from an *ectopic* atrial focus). The QRS complex of a PAC will typically be *narrow* and similar in appearance to normally conducted beats. This is because once the premature impulse arrives at the AV node- it will then be conducted in normal fashion (*Figure B below*)- *unless* conditions for aberrant conduction or bundle branch block are present.

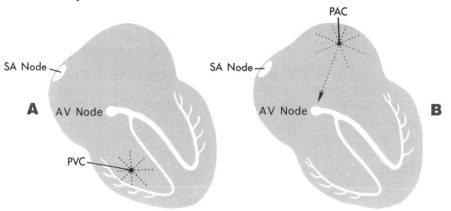

PJCs are *early* occurring beats that arise from the AV node itself. From there, PJCs then follow the path of normal conduction (i.e., over the bundle of His- and into the bundle branch system). As a result, the QRS complex of a PJC should be *narrow* and similar in appearance to the QRS complex of normal sinus beats. P wave polarity may manifest any of the patterns shown on page 143.

PVCs are *early* occurring beats that arise from an ectopic focus from within the *ventricles*. The QRS complex will therefore be *wide* and look very different from the QRS complex of normally conducted beats. Because the ectopic origin of a PVC is *below* the AV node (by definition)- the QRS complex is *not* preceded by a premature P wave (*Figure A above*).

PACs

- Diagnostic Features/Clinical Significance -

Use the **4 *Question Approach*** to interpret the rhythm shown below.

> HINT- Begin your analysis by focusing on the first 3 beats in the tracing to determine the *underlying* rhythm. Then turn your attention to the remaining beats and assess their timing- QRS morphology- and the presence and nature of atrial activity.

Lead II

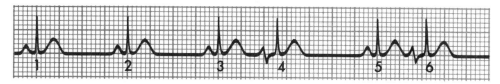

Additional Question:

1. Why do the P waves that precede beats #4 and #6 look different from other P waves on the tracing?

Interpretation:

Applying the **4 Question Approach** to the tracing that appears on page 155- it should be immediately apparent that the rhythm is *not* regular. In this situation- when the pattern of rhythm regularity changes- the *KEY* to interpretaton lies with determining whether there is an *underlying* pattern of regularity for at least a *portion* of the rhythm strip (as we suggest in the **Pearl** on page 152).

The *KEY* to interpreting the tracing that appears on page 155 lies with recognizing that the first 3 beats are regular. The QRS complex for each of these beats is *narrow*- and each QRS is preceded by a *normal* appearing (i.e., *upright*) P wave in this standard lead II monitoring lead. Thus, a **normal sinus rhythm (NSR)** is present for the first 3 beats on the tracing- and this is the *underlying* rhythm!

With this in mind- it should be clear that beats #4 and #6 occur *early*. The QRS complex of these premature beats is narrow and normal in appearance (i.e., virtually identical to the QRS of the sinus-conducted beats). Note that beats #4 and #6 are each preceded by a *premature* P wave. These beats must therefore be **PACs**. The reason the P waves that precede beats #4 and #6 look different from normal sinus P waves is that their site of origin is from an *ectopic* atrial focus (i.e., an atrial site *other than* the SA node). The complete interpretation of this tracing is therefore **sinus rhythm** *with* **PACs**.

Clinical Notes → The importance of PACs depends on the clinical setting in which they occur. PACs are commonly seen in otherwise healthy individuals who do not have underlying heart disease. Even when they occur in patients who do have associated heart disease- they usually do *not* require treatment with antiarrhythmic drugs (unless they are exceedingly frequent and/or associated with severe symptoms). Optimal management of patients with PACs lies with prevention- which may be achieved if a *precipitating* cause (i.e., excessive use of caffeine, alcohol, stimulant drugs, etc.) can be identified and corrected.

PJCs

- Diagnostic Features/Clinical Significance -

Use the **4 *Question Approach*** to interpret the rhythm shown below.

> HINT- Begin your analysis by focusing on the first 3 beats in the tracing
> to determine the *underlying* rhythm. Then turn your attention to the
> remaining beats and assess their timing- QRS morphology- and the
> presence and nature of atrial activity.

Lead II

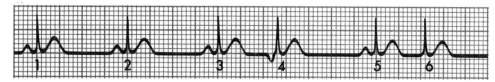

Additional Question:

1. Why does the P wave that precedes beats #4 look different
from other P waves on the tracing? Why is no P wave at
all associated with beat #6?

Interpretation:

As was the case for the rhythm that appeared on page 155- the rhythm on page 157 is also *not* regular. Once again, the *KEY* lies with determining the *underlying* pattern of the rhythm- which is evident from assessment of the first 3 beats. These first 3 beats are regular- with a *narrow* QRS that is preceded by an *upright* P wave with a fixed PR interval. Thus once again, the underlying rhythm is **normal sinus rhythm (NSR)**.

As was the case on page 155- beats #4 and #6 on page 157 both occur *early*. The QRS complex for each of these premature beats is narrow and normal in appearance (i.e., virtually identical to the QRS of the sinus-conducted beats). Note that beat #4 is preceded by a *negatively* directed *premature* P wave. We therefore interpret this beat as a **PJC**- with a pattern of P wave polarity (i.e., negative P wave *preceding* the QRS) that corresponds to Complex B on page 143.

In contrast, no P wave at all is associated with the other early occurring beat on this tracing (i.e., beat #6). Beat #6 is also a **PJC**- in this case with a pattern of P wave polarity that corresponds to Complex C on page 143. The complete interpretation for the rhythm that appears on page 143 is therefore **sinus rhythm** *with* **PJCs**.

Clinical Notes → Technically speaking- it is *not* possible to determine with certainty whether beat #4 on page 157 is truly a PJC- or a PAC arising from an ectopic site that is situated very low down in the atria (i.e., close to the AV node). Fortunately (as emphasized in the Note on page 146)- making this distinction is clinically unimportant- since the clinical significance of PJCs is virtually *identical* to the clinical significance of PACs. Practically speaking- it is well to remember that PACs tend to be much more common than PJCs.

Practice: *Blocked or Aberrant PACs?*

Premature supraventricular beats (i.e., PACs or PJCs) are *not* always conducted to the ventricles- as illustrated in tracings **A** and **B** that appear below.

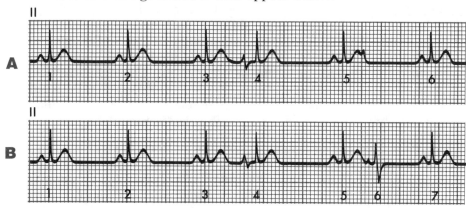

KEY Questions:

1. Can you explain why the premature P wave that immediately follows beat #5 in **Tracing A** is *not* followed by a QRS complex?

HINT- The premature P wave that follows beat #5 in this tracing occurs *so early-* that it is partially hidden by (and produces a notch in) the T wave of beat #5.

2. In **Tracing B**- despite the fact that beat #6 *is* a PAC (i.e., beat #6 is clearly *preceded* by a *premature* P wave)- the QRS complex of this beat is wide and looks different than the QRS of other beats. *Why might this be?*

- 159 -

Answer:

The first 3 beats in each tracing on page 159 are *regular*- with a *narrow* QRS that is preceded by an *upright* P wave with a fixed PR interval. Thus, the *underlying* rhythm for each tracing is **normal sinus rhythm**.

Beat #4 in **_Tracing A_** is clearly a PAC. This beat occurs early- its QRS complex is narrow and normal appearing- and it is *preceded* by a different looking *premature* P wave. A second PAC is seen to occur on this tracing at an even *earlier* point in the cardiac cycle- notching the T wave of beat #5. The reason this P wave is *not* followed by a QRS complex is that it occurs *so early* that it arrives at the AV node at a time *before* recovery (i.e., *repolarization*) of the ventricular conduction system has been completed. As a result, this PAC encounters the ventricles in an *ABSOLUTE refractory state*- at which time conduction of the premature impulse *beyond* the AV node is simply *not* possible (i.e., this **PAC** is **"blocked"**).

In **_Tracing B_**- *on page 159* beat #4 is again a PAC. Beat #6 in this tracing also occurs early- and manifests a QRS complex that is wider and different appearing than the QRS complex of other beats. Nevertheless, beat #6 in Tracing B on page 159 *is* preceded by a *premature* P wave- which means that this beat must also be a PAC! The reason its QRS complex looks different is that this **PAC** is *conducted* with **aberration**. Note how this PAC occurs at a slightly *later* point in the cardiac cycle than the PAC that follows the T wave of beat #5 in Tracing A. Presumably, this second PAC in Tracing B occurs during the *RELATIVE refractory period*- at a time when the ventricular conduction system has only *partially* recovered- and is therefore *not yet able* to allow normal conduction. QRS widening and the altered (i.e., *aberrant*) QRS appearance of beat #6 in Tracing B reflect conduction delay that results from *refractoriness* in at least one of the bundle branches or conduction fascicles.

Note ➔ It would be ever so easy in Tracing A to overlook the premature P wave that notches the T wave of beat #5- especially if one failed to compare the normally *smooth* T wave configuration of all other beats on this tracing with this T wave. It might be equally easy to overlook the premature P wave that precedes beat #6 in Tracing B (and to mistake this wider, different appearing QRS complex for a PVC)- if one failed to appreciate that the *ever-so-tiny* notch that precedes this QRS complex is in fact a PAC.

PVCs

- Diagnostic Features/Clinical Significance -

Use the *4 Question Approach* to interpret the rhythm shown below.

> HINT- Begin your analysis by focusing on the first 3 beats in the tracing to determine the *underlying* rhythm. Then turn your attention to the remaining beats and assess their timing- QRS morphology- and the presence (or absence) of associated atrial activity.

Lead II

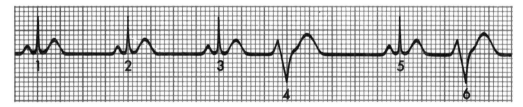

Additional Question:

1. Why do the QRS complexes of beats #4 and #6 look so different from other QRS complexes on the tracing?

Interpretation:

The rhythm that appears on page 161 is similar to the rhythms shown on pages 155, 157, and 159- in that the first 3 beats in each of these tracings are *regular* and sinus-conducted. Thereafter, a number of *early* beats occur.

Beats #4 and #6 on page 161 occur early. The QRS complex of these premature beats is markedly widened and very different in appearance from the sinus-conducted beats. There is no premature P wave associated with either widened complex. Thus, beats #4 and #6 on page 161 *must* be PVCs. Complete interpretation of this tracing would therefore be **sinus rhythm** *with* **PVCs**.

<u>**Clinical Notes**</u> → The occurrence of premature beats is exceedingly common in clinical practice- especially in acute care situations. Practically speaking- primary goals of the emergency care provider should be twofold:

1. To determine the *type* of premature beat (i.e., PVC- or PAC/PJC).
2. To evaluate the **clinical setting** in which the premature beats occur.

Clinically, the importance of distinguishing between PVCs and PACs or PJCs- is that PVCs are much more likely to warrant specific treatment. This is particularly true when the ventricular ectopy occurs in an emergency situation. Thus, the occurrence of **new-onset PVCs** in a patient with acute ischemic heart disease and/or acute myocardial infarction mandates concern because of the risk that it may precipitate a potentially *life-threatening* ventricular arrhythmia (such as ventricular tachycardia or fibrillation)- especially if the new-onset ventricular ectopy is *frequent* and *repetitive* forms are noted (*See pages 167-170*).

In contrast, the occurrence of either PACs or PJCs in an identical situation would be of far less concern- and would therefore be much less likely to warrant treatment- especially if the patientt remained asymptomatic.

Practice: *PACs, PVCs- or both?*

Use the **4 Question Approach** to interpret the rhythm shown below.

> HINT- Begin your analysis with an overall survey of the tracing for regularity- or at least for *portions* of the tracing with regularity. Then look to determine the *underlying* rhythm.

Lead II

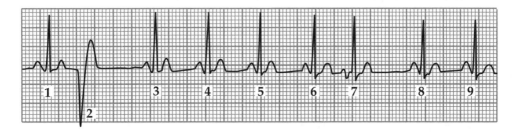

Interpretation:

The rhythm that appears on page 163 is *not* completely regular. Nevertheless, the *underlying* rhythm appears to be **sinus**- as evidenced by inspection of beats #3 through #6. During this segment of the rhythm strip, the R-R interval is regular- the QRS complex is narrow- and each QRS is preceded by a normal appearing (i.e., *upright*) P wave in this lead II monitoring lead.

Two beats interrupt the underlying pattern of regularity: beat #2 and beat #7. Both of these beats occur *earlier* than expected (in view of the underlying rhythm):

> **Beat #2**- is wide- very different in appearance from other QRS complexes on the tracing- and is *not* preceded by a premature P wave. This beat is a **PVC**.

> **Beat #7**- is narrow and virtually *identical* in appearance to the QRS complex of other sinus-conducted beats. Beat #7 must therefore be a premature *SUPRAventricular* impulse (i.e., *either* a PAC or a PJC). The fact that this beat is preceded by a premature P wave that is *not* inverted in this standard lead II is evidence that this early beat is a **PAC**.

Complete interpretation of the rhythm that appears on page 163 would therefore be **sinus rhythm** *with a* **PAC** *and a* **PVC**.

> **PEARL** → Premature beats (i.e., PACs, PJCs, and PVCs) alter the underlying pattern of rhythm regularity by their early occurrence. As a result of an early beat- the ensuing R-R interval is likely to be prolonged until the underlying pattern of regularity can be reestablished. This explains why a slight pause is seen following beats #2 and #7 in the tracing on page 163.
>
> Finally- we draw attention to the fact that the premature P wave preceding beat #7 on page 163 is clearly *different* in appearance from the P wave preceding each of the sinus-conducted beats (i.e., this P wave is *biphasic*- whereas the P waves of sinus beats on this tracing are upright *without* any terminal negative deflection). The presence of a different appearing P wave is further support of a different (i.e., *ectopic*) atrial site of origin for this PAC.

<u>Practice</u>: *PACs, PVCs- or both?*

Use the **4 *Question Approach*** to interpret the rhythm shown below.

> <u>HINT #1</u>- Begin your analysis with an overall survey of the tracing for reg-
> ularity- or at least for *portions* of the tracing with regularity. Then look
> to determine the *underlying* rhythm.

> <u>HINT #2</u>- Save analysis of the most *abnormal* appearing beat (i.e., beat #3)
> for last. Be sure to look *carefully* at the T wave *preceding* this beat-
> *before* deciding on whether to call this beat a PAC or PVC.

Lead MCL$_6$

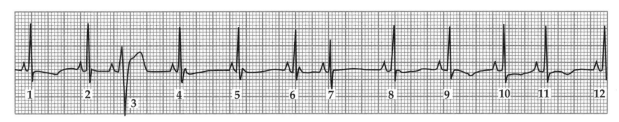

<u>Additional Question</u> → Can sinus rhythm be diagnosed
despite the fact that a lead *other than* lead II is being monitored?

Interpretation:

An extremely helpful principal for rhythm interpretation was introduced in the Pearl on page 152:

> When a rhythm strip contains information that is *easy* to evaluate- *as well as* information that is more difficult to evaluate- **begin *first* with that part of the tracing that is *easiest* to interpret.** *Save the more difficult part(s) for last.*

The reason we suggest saving analysis of beat #3 on page 165 for last is that assessment of this beat is the most problematic part of the rhythm. What is clear- is that the overall rhythm in this tracing is *not* regular. However, despite this irregularity- attention to beats #1-2, #4-6, #8-10, and #12- indicates that the *underlying* rhythm is once again **sinus**. That is, the R-R interval for beats included within each of these short segments is constant- the QRS complex remains consistently narrow- and each QRS is preceded by a similar appearing P wave with a fixed PR interval. Thus, even though this rhythm strip is *not* obtained from lead II- the presence of consistant P wave morphology and the constant PR interval strongly suggest that the rhythm is sinus.

Beats #3, #7, and #11 all occur early. The latter two beats are clearly PACs- since each is preceded by a premature P wave and associated with a narrow QRS complex that looks very similar to that of the sinus-conducted beats.

Beat #3 is also a PAC. Despite the fact that the QRS complex of this beat is wider and different in morphology- it is clearly preceded by a *premature* P wave. The reason this QRS looks different is that this PAC is conducted with aberration (*See pages 159-160*). Complete interpretation of this rhythm would therefore be **sinus rhythm** *with* **PACs-** *some of which are conducted with* **aberration***.*

> **PEARL (Beyond the Core)** → Close inspection of the QRS complex of beat #7 on page 165 reveals that the morphology of this beat *also* differs (albeit ever so slightly) from the QRS morphology of normally conducted beats (i.e., the R wave is not quite as tall- and the S wave is slightly deeper). It is therefore likely that beat #7 is also conducted with at least some degree of aberrant conduction.

Repetitive Forms of PVCs

The term *repetitive* PVCs- is used to describe the occurrence of *more* than one PVC in a row. Examples of repetitive forms of ventricular ectopy include:

- *Ventricular COUPLETS-* when 2 PVCs occur in a row.

- *Ventricular SALVOS-* when 3 PVCs occur in a row. By definition, the occurrence of 3 or more PVCs in a row constitutes **ventricular tachycardia (VT).**

Lead II

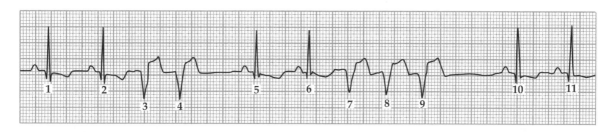

Questions → Is the *underlying* rhythm in the above tracing sinus? Which beats make up the ventricular *couplet* ? Which beats make up the *salvo* ?

Interpretation:

The easiest way to interpret the rhythm that appears on page 167 is:

1. To initially *ignore* the abnormal looking beats (i.e., beats #3-4; and #7-8-9).
2. To determine the *underlying* rhythm.
3. To return to the abnormal looking beats.

Although the overall rhythm that appears on page 167 is clearly *not* regular- inspection of beats #1-2; #5-6; and #10-11- suggests that the *underlying* rhythm is once again **sinus**. We arrive at this conclusion because the QRS complex for each of these beats is narrow, and a normal appearing (i.e., *upright*) P wave precedes each QRS complex with a constant PR interval. The underlying rate of this sinus rhythm appears to be about **85 beats/minute**- as evidenced by the fact that the R-R interval for each of the pairs of beats noted above is constant and *between* 3 to 4 large boxes in duration.

Beats #3, 4, 7, 8, and 9 are all **PVCs**. Each of these beats is wide and bizarre in appearance- and *none* of these beats are preceded by a premature P wave. As defined on the preceding page- beats #3-4 constitute a ***ventricular COUPLET***- and beats #7-8-9 constitute a ***ventricular SALVO***.

Clinical Notes → As alluded to on page 162- PVCs are cause for concern when they are frequent and when *repetitive* forms (i.e., couplets, salvos- and longer runs of VT) are noted. This is especially true when such PVCs are new in onset, and occur in a setting of acute ischemic heart disease or other cardiac emergency.

Multiform PVCs

PVCs may manifest more than a single morphologic appearance in a given patient. When this occurs, PVCs are said to be *"multiform"*.

Lead MCL₁

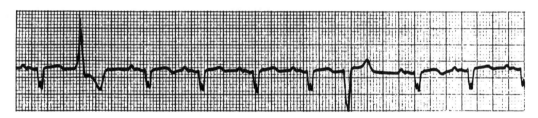

Question → Can you think of 2 reasons why PVCs in the same patient may sometimes look morphologically different?

Interpretation:

The underlying rhythm for the tracing that appears on page 169 is **sinus**- as evidenced by regularity of *most* R-R intervals and the presence of a normal appearing (albeit small) upright P wave with a fixed PR interval in this lead MCL$_1$ monitoring lead. The PR interval associated with each sinus-conducted beat is at the upper limit of normal (i.e., approximately 1 large box- or 0.20 second in duration). QRS interval duration is also at the upper limit of normal (i.e., about half a large box- or 0.10 second in duration).

There are 2 abnormal appearing beats on this tracing. Both are wide- and neither is preceded by a premature P wave. This suggests that these early occurring beats are both **PVCs**. The first PVC manifests an entirely upright (i.e., R wave) configuration- whereas the second PVC manifests an entirely negative (i.e., a QS) configuration. Thus, complete interpretation of the rhythm that appears on page 169 would be **sinus rhythm** *with* **multiform PVCs.**

In the past, PVCs of differing morphologies were said to be *multifocal*- because it used to be thought that they arose from different ectopic foci. It is now known that this is *not* necessarily the case. PVCs may arise from the *same* focus- but use a *different* reentrant pathway (in the course of their travel through ventricular myocardium). This may result in a very different morphologic appearance for two PVCs- despite the fact that they arise from the same ventricular ectopic focus. It would seem more appropriate to refer to such different appearing PVCs as *"multiform"*- rather than multifocal.

Clinical Notes → A fact that is still *not* well appreciated by many health care providers is that many (if not most) patients who have frequent PVCs- will *also* have multiform PVCs. Fortunately, the presence of *multiformity* per se is *not* nearly as ominous as used to be thought. Of much greater concern than the finding of multiform PVCs are *repetitive* PVCs (i.e., ventricular couplets, salvos- and longer runs of VT)- since this is what predisposes susceptible patients to develop sustained VT/V Fib!

Bi- Tri- **and** Quadrigeminy

At times, a *regularly* occurring pattern of PVCs may be present- in which every *second- third-* or *fourth* beat may be a PVC. The following terminology is used to describe these patterns:

- ■ *Ventricular BIGEMINY*- when every *second* beat is a PVC.

  - ■ *Ventricular TRIGEMINY*- when every *third* beat is a PVC.

    - ■ *Ventricular QUADRIGEMINY*- when every *fourth* beat is a PVC.

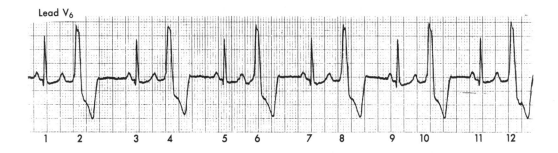

Questions → Which regularly occurring pattern of PVCs is seen in the above tracing? What is the *underlying* rhythm?

Interpretation:

The underlying rhythm for the tracing that appears on page 171 is **sinus**- as evidenced by beats #1, 3, 5, 7, 9, and 11. The QRS complex for each of these beats is narrow and normal appearing, and each QRS is preceded by a similar looking upright P wave with a constant (and normal) PR interval. Thus, despite the fact that a lead *other than* lead II is being used for monitoring- and despite the variation in QRS morphology that is seen on this tracing- recognition of an underlying sinus mechanism is still possible.

Every other beat on this tracing is widened (i.e., beats #2, 4, 6, 8, 10, and 12 are all clearly more than half a large box in duration). QRS morphology of these widened beats is markedly different from the QRS morphology of sinus-conducted beats (i.e., sinus beats manifest a qR configuration- whereas the widened beats consist of a single upright deflection in the form of a monophasic R wave). Premature P waves do *not* appear to precede the widened beats. It is therefore most likely that every other beat on this tracing is a **PVC**- which means that the rhythm is *ventricular BIGEMINY*.

Note that although we *are* able to establish the presence of *underlying* sinus rhythm in this tracing- we are *not* able to determine the underlying sinus rate. This is because there is simply no place on the tracing where two normal (i.e., sinus-conducted) beats occur in a row. As a result- description of the rhythm as *ventricular bigeminy* is all that need be said.

Clinical Notes → The significance of *ventricular bigeminy* is similar to the significance of the finding of frequent (but *non-repetitive*) PVCs. As emphasized on page 162 the most important factor (*by far!*) in assessing the significance of PVCs is the clinical setting in which they occur. Development of *new-onset* ventricular bigeminy in a patient with acute ischemic heart disease might therefore be cause for concern. On the other hand- recognition of *long-standing* ventricular bigeminy in an *asymptomatic* patient who does *not* have underlying heart disease- is definitely NOT an emergency (and may not require any intervention at all)!

Practice: *What is the rhythm?*

Use the **4 Question Approach** to interpret the rhythm shown below.

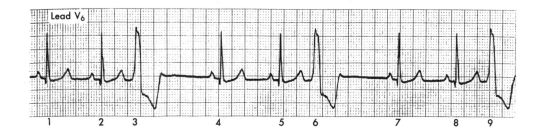

Questions:

1. Is there a *pattern* to the occurrence of the wider beats?

> HINT- The above tracing was obtained in *follow-up* from the same
> patient whose rhythm was shown on page 171. *Feel free to refer to
> pages 171-172 in formulating your response.*

2. Is the *underlying* rhythm for the above tracing sinus? If so-
what is the underlying sinus rate?

Interpretation:

The rhythm that appears on page 173 is *not* regular. Nevertheless, the *underlying* rhythm is still **sinus**- as evidenced by beats #1-2; #4-5; and #7-8. The QRS complex for all of these beats is narrow- and each QRS is preceded by a similar looking upright P wave with a constant (and normal) PR interval. The underlying rate of this sinus rhythm varies slightly- as determined by the fact that the R-R interval for each of the pairs of sinus beats is *between* 4 and 5 large boxes in duration. The heart rate is therefore *between* **65-70 beats/minute**. (It is difficult to tell from this short rhythm strip if the underlying sinus rate varies enough to qualify the rhythm as sinus "arrhythmia"- *See Note on page 100*).

The most remarkable finding of the tracing on page 173 is that evey *third* beat is widened (i.e., beats #3, 6, and 9 are all clearly *more* than half a large box in duration). As was the case for the widened beats on page 171- QRS morphology for the widened beats on this tracing differs greatly from QRS morphology of the sinus-conducted beats. Premature P waves do *not* precede the widened beats. Thus, every *third* beat on this tracing is a **PVC**- and the rhythm is *ventricular TRIGEMINY*.

PEARL (Beyond the Core) → Return for a moment to the rhythm that appears on page 171. Because one *never* sees two sinus-conducted beats in a row on that tracing- it is impossible to know whether or not a premature P wave might be buried *within* the T wave that precedes each PVC. That is, one can *not* be certain what a "normal" T wave *should* look like- which makes it impossible to know if the T waves on that tracing are naturally peaked- or are "being peaked" by subtly concealed PACs.

    A *follow-up* tracing on that patient appears on page 173- and resolves the problem. Consecutive sinus beats now *are* seen (i.e., beats #1-2; #4-5; and #7-8 on page 173). The occurrence of two sinus beats in a row allows us to determine the appearance of a "normal" T wave (i.e., the T wave of beats #1, 4, and 7). Because this "normal" T wave is *identical* in appearance to the T wave that precedes each widened complex- we can be much more confident of our conclusion that premature P waves do *not* precede beats #3, 6, and 9 on page 173- *and that these premature beats MUST therefore be PVCs.*

Practice: *What is the rhythm?*

Use the **4 Question Approach** to interpret the rhythm shown below.

> <u>HINT</u>- Save interpretation of the most *abnormal* looking beats (i.e., beats #4 and #9) for last.

Lead II

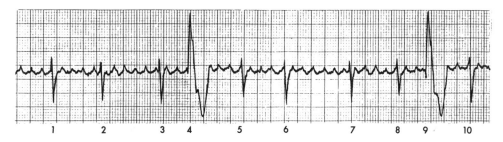

Question → Is the *underlying* rhythm sinus?

Interpretation:

The easiest way to approach interpretation of the rhythm that appears on page 175 is to initially *ignore* the two abnormal looking beats (i.e., beats #4 and #9). Inspection of the rest of the tracing suggests that the underlying rhythm is *not* sinus (since normal sinus P waves are *not* seen). Instead there is an *irregular irregularity* to the rhythm. Fairly regular atrial activity *is* present- in the form of a *sawtooth* pattern that occurs at a rate that is *close* to **300/minute** (i.e., atrial spikes are noted at an interval of *just under* 1 large box in duration). This suggests that the *underlying* rhythm is ***atrial flutter***- in this case with a ***variable (****albeit controlled****)* ventricular response**.

Return to the two *abnormal* looking beats on this tracing (i.e., beats #4 and #9 on page 175). Both of these complexes are wide- bizarre in appearance- and markedly different in configuration from the other beats on this tracing. Premature P waves do *not* precede either of these wide beats. They *can't*- since the underlying rhythm is atrial flutter (which by definition *excludes* the possibility of *premature* atrial activity). Thus, the widened beats *must* be **PVCs**. Complete interpretation of the rhythm is therefore- *atrial flutter* with *variable* AV conduction- and *PVCs*.

> **Comment** → Note how interpretation of this rhythm is facilitated by applying the principal that was introduced on page 168:
>
> - Initially *ignore* the abnormal looking beats.
> - Determine the *underlying* rhythm.
> - Then return to interpret the abnormal looking beats.

Clinical Notes → As emphasized on page 118- the most common ventricular response to atrial flutter (*by far!*)- is with 2:1 AV conduction. The next most common response is with 4:1 AV conduction. Odd conduction ratios (i.e., 1:1, 3:1, 5:1, etc.) are rare. On occasion, atrial flutter may present with *variable* AV conduction- as it does for the rhythm that appears on the page 175. As might be imagined, distinction between atrial flutter and atrial fibrillation may be difficult in such cases- especially if flutter activity is not well seen in the lead being monitored.

VT

- *Ventricular Tachycardia* -

On page 167 we defined *ventricular tachycardia (VT)* as the presence of 3 or more PVCs in a row. There are 2 types of VT:

- **NON-Sustained VT**- when the run of VT is *short-lived* (i.e., usually *less* than 30 seconds in duration).

- **SUSTAINED VT**- when the run of VT persists.

Lead II

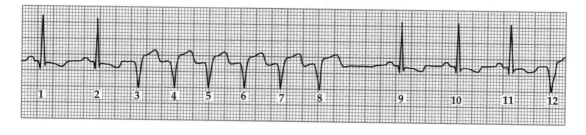

Questions → What type of VT is seen in the above rhythm? What is the heart rate *during* the tachycardia?

Interpretation:

As on previous tracings- the easiest way to approach interpretation of the rhythm that appears on the page 177 is to initially *ignore* the run of abnormal looking beats. Instead, focus first on the *normal* appearing beats- and try to determine the *underlying* rhythm. The normal appearing beats on this tracing are beats #1, 2, 9, 10, and 11. The QRS complex for each of these beats is narrow- and normal sinus P waves (i.e., *upright* in lead II) precede each QRS with a constant (and normal) PR interval. Thus, the *underlying* rhythm is **sinus**. Since the R-R interval *between* sinus beats is between 3 and 4 large boxes in duration- the underlying sinus rate is about **85 beats/minute**.

Sinus rhythm is *interrupted* on this tracing by a 6-beat run of tachycardia (i.e., beats #3 through #8). QRS complexes during this run are *wide*- and *not* associated with atrial activity. This suggests that the 6-beat run represents an episode of **NON-sustained VT**. Following this run, a short *pause* ensues (i.e., the period *between* beats #8 and #9)- after which sinus rhythm resumes. The last beat on the tracing (i.e., beat #12) is another PVC.

> **Comment** → In addition to noting the *onset- duration-* and *manner of termination* of a tachycardia- full description also entails determination of its *regularity* and *rate*. The R-R interval separating widened beats in this example is regular and between 2 to 3 large boxes in duration. Since it is slightly closer to the former- we estimate heart rate *during* the tachycardia to be *about* 130 beats/minute.
>
> **Clinical Note** → The rhythm that appears on page 177 was obtained as a *follow-up* tracing on the same patient whose rhythm was shown on page 167. It illustrates how the presence of *repetitive* PVCs (*that were seen on the earlier tracing*) may sometimes forebode development of longer runs of VT.

VT

- Ventricular Tachycardia -

As noted on page 177- there are 2 principal types of VT: 1) ***NON-sustained VT*** ; and 2) ***Sustained VT***. Which of these two types is illustrated by the rhythm shown below?

Lead II

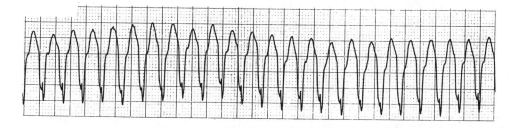

<u>Additional Questions:</u>

1. Are you *sure* that the above rhythm is really VT? *What else might this rhythm be ?*

2. When doubt exists about the etiology of a ***WIDE-complex*** **tachycardia-** what should you assume until *proven* otherwise?

Interpretation:

The easiest way to interpret the rhythm that appears on page 179 is to apply the **4 Question Approach** :

    i) The QRS complex is *wide*. Although it is admittedly difficult to determine the precise point at which the QRS complex begins and the point at which it ends- it seems certain that the QRS complex is at the very least *more* than *half* a large box in duration.

    ii) The rhythm is *regular.* The R-R interval is between 1 and 2 large boxes in duration. Use of the **'Every OTHER Beat' Method** facilitates estimation of heart rate. As described on pages 55-58- the method works by first calculating the heart rate of every *other* beat (i.e., *half* the rate). Then *double* this number. The R-R interval of every *other* beat for the tracing on page 179 is just *under* 3 large boxes in duration. Thus- *half* the rate is about 115 beats/minute. The *actual* rate is therefore about **230 beats/ minute** (i.e., 115 X 2).

    iii) & iv) There are no P waves (or other signs of atrial activity).

Comment → The rhythm that appears on page 179 is described as a regular **WIDE-complex tachycardia**. As noted above, the heart rate for the rhythm is 230 beats/minute- and there is no evidence of atrial activity. Although it is possible that the etiology of this rhythm could be *SUPRAventricular* (with QRS widening as the result of *either* preexisting bundle branch block *or* aberrant conduction)-**Ventricular Tachycardia** <u>must</u> be assumed until proven otherwise !

    On page 177 we defined **sustained VT** as *persistence* of this rhythm- usually for a period of *more* than 30 seconds. It is important to appreciate that despite the *appearance* of being "sustained"- the rhythm strip shown on page 179 lasts for *only* 6.2 seconds! Perception of time duration may be deceptive during an emergency situation- *so that time seems often to "expand" in such settings.*

Causes of a Regular <u>WCT</u>
- (<u>W</u>IDE-<u>C</u>omplex <u>T</u>achycardia) -

A common and extremely important diagnostic problem in emergency cardiac care is to determine the cause of a regular <u>**W**</u>*ide-*<u>**C**</u>*omplex* <u>**T**</u>*achycardia* **(WCT)**. There are 5 principal entities to consider:

<u>Causes of a Regular WCT (When the Etiology is Uncertain)</u> :
>   1. Ventricular Tachycardia
>   2. *Ventricular Tachycardia*
>   3. *VENTRICULAR TACHYCARDIA*
>   4. SVT with aberration
>   5. SVT with *pre-existing* bundle branch block (BBB)

Lead II

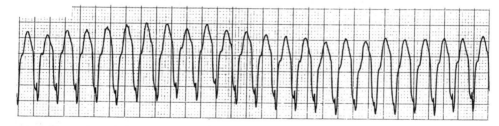

<u>KEY Questions:</u>

1. Why do you suppose we list VT as the first 3 causes to consider?

2. Should you be dissuaded from considering VT for the rhythm shown above if the patient in question was *alert- asymptomatic-* and *normotensive* ?

The Regular WCT of Uncertain Etiology

There are two major reasons for listing VT as the first *three* entities to consider in the differential diagnosis of a **WIDE-Complex Tachycardia (WCT)**. They are:

1. The fact that *by far* (!)- VT is the most common cause of a *WIDE-complex* tachycardia when the rhythm is *regular* (or at least *fairly* regular)- and when normal sinus P waves are nowhere to be seen.

2. VT is generally a much more *serious* rhythm disorder than SVT- and it is often potentially life-threatening (with high risk of deteriorating to ventricular fibrillation). In contrast, abrupt hemodynamic decompensation is much less likely to occur in association with supraventricular tachyarrhythmias. Emphasizing the need to *always* consider VT- *until PROVEN otherwise* (as we do by repetition in our differential list)- minimizes the chance of missing the diagnosis of VT.

PEARLS in ECG Diagnosis → The topic of evaluating a *WCT* and distinguishing between VT and SVT with aberrant conduction or preexisting BBB is an extensive one. We therefore devote an entire section to this in the *advanced* portion of this book (**Section 2B**- beginning on page 315) and restrict our comments here to the following *KEY* points:

- When *doubt* exists about the etiology of a WCT- *assume VT.* Doing so prevents overlooking this potentially life-threatening arrhythmia. Practically speaking, you will be correct *most* of the time- since VT is so much more common than SVT with either aberrant conduction or preexisting BBB. VT is especially likely to be the cause of a WCT when the patient is an *older* adult who has a history of underlying heart disease!

- VT will still be the most likely diagnosis- even when the patient is *alert-asymptomatic-* and *normotensive*! It is important to appreciate that some patients may tolerate sustained VT *surprisingly* well- and maintain consciousness despite persistence of this rhythm for *long* periods of time (i.e., of hours- *or even days!*).

Practice: *What is the rhythm?*

The tracing below was obtained from an elderly man with a history of a myocardial infarction in the past. He was awake and alert with a BP = 150/80 mm Hg at the time this tracing was recorded.

Lead II

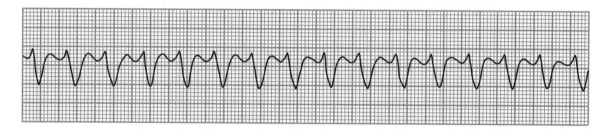

Questions:

1. What 5 diagnostic possibilities should be considered in your differential diagnosis for the tracing shown above?

    HINT- Feel free to refer to page 181 in formulating your answer.

2. Should this patient's clinical presentation (i.e., the fact that the patient was alert and normotensive)- affect your answer?

Interpretation:

Applying the **4 *Question Approach*** to the rhythm that appears on page 183- we note the following:

  i) The QRS complex is markedly *widened*. Although admittedly difficult to determine the point at which the S wave (of the QRS) ends and the ST segment begins- it seems certain that the QRS complex during this tachycardia must be *at least* 0.12 second in duration (if not considerably longer).

  ii) The rhythm is *regular*. The R-R interval is approximately 2 large boxes in duration- so that the heart rate is close to **150 beats/minute**.

  iii) & iv) There are no P waves (or other signs of atrial activity).

> **Comment** → Use of the *4 Question Approach* defines the rhythm on page 183 as a regular **WIDE-complex tachycardia**. Atrial activity is absent. As noted on page 181- the principal entities to consider in the differential diagnosis include:
>
>   1. VT
>   2. VT
>   3. VT
>   4. SVT with aberration
>   5. SVT with preexisting BBB

> Clearly- **VT must be assumed until *proven* otherwise!** The fact that this patient was alert and hemodynamically stable at the time the ECG was recorded is encouraging from a clinical perspective- *but should do nothing to dissuade you from assuming VT (until proven otherwise)*. VT is especially likely to be the diagnosis in this case in view of this patient's clinical history (i.e., the fact that the patient is an *older* adult with a history of *underlying* heart disease).

What if you *think* that
the rhythm *is* VT?

On page 184- we emphasized the need to assume VT for the rhythm shown below- *until proven otherwise.* Working on this assumption (i.e., that you *think* the rhythm is VT)- and given that the tracing was obtained from an elderly man who at the time was awake, alert, and normotensive- *how should you proceed clinically?*

Lead II

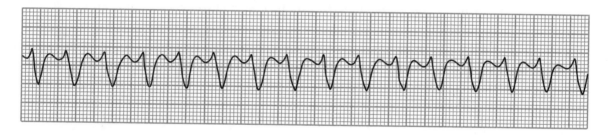

Questions:

1. What diagnostic/therapeutic interventions might be indicated?

2. What would you do if this patient suddenly decompensated and became hypotensive? If he became unresponsive and the pulse was lost?

When you think the rhythm is VT

The *KEY* to management of **sustained VT** lies with determining the patient's hemodynamic status. There are **3** possibilities:

1. *There is* **NO pulse.** This defines the condition known as **pulseless VT**. The patient will die unless *immediate* action is taken. The treatment recommended is the *same* as for ventricular fibrillation (V Fib)- immediate *unsynchronized* countershock (i.e., defibrillation) with 200-360 joules.

2. A pulse *IS* present- *but the patient is* **UNSTABLE.** Hemodynamic instability may be reflected by hypotension, a change in mental status, chest pain, and/or shortness of breath. Treatment is *urgently* needed- but there will usually be time to apply *synchronized* cardioversion. By setting the defibrillator to deliver the electrical impulse at the least "vulnerable" point in the cardiac cycle (i.e., on the upstroke of the R wave)- the chance of inadvertently precipitating V Fib with synchronized cardioversion is minimized.

3. A pulse *IS* present- *but the patient is* **hemodynamically STABLE.** As emphasized in the pearls on page 182- some patients tolerate sustained VT *surprisingly* well- and maintain consciousness (*despite* persistence of this rhythm) for *long* periods of time (i.e., of hours- *or even days!*). As a result, you will usually have time to:

   - *Catch YOUR breath*!
   - Consider additional diagnostic measures (*if/as* needed) to verify the diagnosis (i.e., obtaining a 12-lead ECG *during* the tachycardia, comparing the current rhythm to *prior* tracings, etc.).
   - Initiate a trial of medical therapy (i.e., with lidocaine, procainamide- or other antiarrhythmic drugs).
   - Remain *ever ready* to cardiovert the patient- should hemodynamic decompensation occur at *any* time during the treatment process.

PEARL → Realize that you will *not* always know for sure what the true diagnosis of a WCT is. *Even the experts DON'T always know!*

<u>Practice</u>: *What is the rhythm?*

HINT- Despite QRS widening- *this rhythm is <u>not</u> VT*!

Use the **4 *Question Approach*** to interpret the rhythm shown below.

Lead II

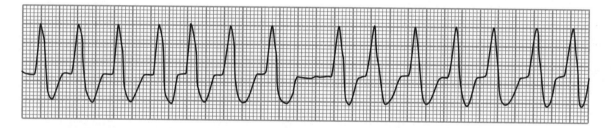

<u>Questions:</u>

1. Given that the above tracing is *not* VT- what then is the *underlying* rhythm?

   <u>HINT</u>- Consider the nature of atrial activity- and the regularity of the rhythm (or rather the *lack* thereof!)- in formulating your answer.

2. Why might the QRS be widened- despite the fact that this rhythm is *not* VT?

Interpretation:

Applying the **4 Question Approach** to the rhythm that appears on page 187- we note the following:

  i) The QRS complex is *wide*. It is clearly *more* than half a large box in duration.

  ii) The rhythm is *irregularly* irregular. R-R intervals *continually* change from one beat to the next *without* any recognizable pattern.

  iii) & iv) There are no P waves (or other signs of atrial activity).

> **Comment** → Despite obvious QRS widening- the rhythm that appears on page 187 is *not* VT. Instead, the *irregular* irregularity of the ventricular response- in conjunction with the *absence* of atrial activity- strongly suggest that the rhythm is **atrial fibrillation (A Fib)**. The ventricular response is described as *moderately* rapid (since most R-R intervals are between 2 and 3 large boxes in duration).
>
> The most likely explanation for QRS widening in this tracing despite the fact that the rhythm is supraventricular- is that this patient must have *preexisting* BBB. Another (albeit somewhat less likely) possibility is that there is *aberrant* conduction.

> **Note** → Distinction between sustained VT and A Fib with QRS widening from preexisting BBB is often difficult. This is especially true when the ventricular response is relatively rapid (as it is here)- since A Fib may *seem* regular when the ventricular response is fast (*See Comment on page 140*).
>
> Although sustained VT is usually a regular rhythm- the ventricular response *may* vary (at least to *some* degree). However, the rhythm will usually *not* be as irregularly irregular as seen on page 187. Further support that this rhythm represents A Fib might be forthcoming if prior tracings were available for comparison (to determine if the A Fib and/or BBB were present in the past).

<u>Practice</u>: *What is the rhythm?*

<u>HINT</u>- Despite QRS widening- *this rhythm is <u>not</u> VT* !

Use the **4 *Question Approach*** to interpret the rhythm shown below.

Lead V$_1$

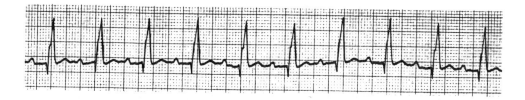

<u>Question:</u>

1. Why might the QRS be widened- despite the fact that this rhythm is *not* VT?

    <u>HINT</u>- What is the *underlying* rhythm?

Interpretation:

Applying the **4 *Question Approach*** to the rhythm that appears on page 189- we note the following:

i) The QRS complex is *wide* (i.e., it is clearly *more* than half a large box in duration).

ii) The rhythm is *regular.* The R-R interval is between 3 and 4 large boxes in duration- so that the heart rate is about **85 beats/minute**.

iii) & iv) Normal appearing P waves are seen preceding each QRS complex with a fixed (albeit slightly prolonged) PR interval (of approximately 0.22 second).

> **Comment** → Despite the fact that a lead *other than* lead II was used for monitoring, it should be clear that the mechanism of the rhythm that appears on page 189 is **sinus**- since regularly occurring P waves precede each QRS with a constant PR interval. As will be discussed in section 1G *(on pages 241-242)*- the PR interval is prolonged (i.e., *more* than 0.20-0.21 second in duration)- which means that **1° AV block** is present. The reason the QRS complex is wide is that the patient has right bundle branch block (RBBB).

Note → The rhythms that are shown on pages 187 and 189 illustrate how QRS widening will *not always* be the result of VT. Clues suggesting a supraventricular etiology are present in each case. The point to emphasize is that VT *becomes* the most common cause of a WCT (*by far!*)- when the rhythm is *regular* and when normal sinus P waves are *absent.*

Section 1E- *Late* Beats/*Escape* Rhythms

Late Beats

We reviewed the concept of *EARLY-* and *LATE-occurring* beats on pages 151-152. The Figure below is reproduced from these pages.

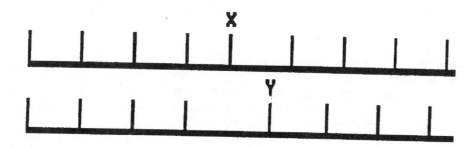

Questions:

1. What is the *overall* pattern of regularity for the two schematic tracings shown above?

2. What is the *relative* timing of the complex labeled " **Y** " compared to the complex labeled " **X** " ?

Answers:

Both of the schematic examples that appear on page 191 exhibit a pattern of underlying *regularity*- with the exception of the beats labeled "X" and "Y" (and the interval that immediately follows these complexes). The complex labeled " **X** " interrupts the pattern by occurring *early*. In contrast- the complex labeled " **Y** " interrupts the pattern by occurring *late*.

Clinical examples of *EARLY-occurring* beats include the 3 types of *premature* complexes (i.e., PACs, PJCs, and PVCs). As discussed on pages 153-162- distinction between these 3 types of premature beats is made by assessing the appearance of the QRS complex and evaluating the nature of associated atrial activity (or the *lack* thereof).

In contrast to premature beats-**LATE**-*occurring* beats most often reflect **"escape"** activity arising from a *lower* pacemaker. Escape beats serve the specific function of *preventing* excessive bradycardia. Diagnostically- the *same* principles used to distinguish between the 3 types of premature beats are also used to surmise the site of the escape pacemaker- except that the *timing* is different:

- *Escape beats arising from the* **Atria**- usually manifest a QRS complex that is *narrow* and similar in appearance to the QRS complex of normally conducted beats. Atrial escape beats are generally preceded by a P wave that should look different from the normal sinus P wave (since by definition, the escape focus is arising from some *other* site in the atria).

- *Escape beats arising from the* **AV Node**- usually also manifest a QRS complex that is *narrow*. Although the QRS complex of junctional escape beats is most often quite similar in appearance to the QRS of normally conducted beats- there may be *slight* differences in QRS morphology (reflecting the fact that these escape beats may arise from different points *within* the AV node itself). Atrial activity associated with junctional escape beats may take on any of the forms illustrated on page 143 (i.e., a *negative* P wave in lead II that either precedes or follows the QRS- or no P wave at all).

- *Escape beats arising from the* **Ventricles**- manifest a QRS complex that is *wide* and very different in appearance from the QRS of normally conducted beats.

Escape Rhythms

The SA node is the principal pacemaker of the heart. With normal sinus rhythm (NSR)- the SA node discharges at a rate of between 60-100 beats/ minute. What would you expect to happen if for some reason the SA node *failed* to initiate the electrical impulse?

> HINT- What other area(s) of the heart (seen in the Figure below) might
> take over the pacemaking function?

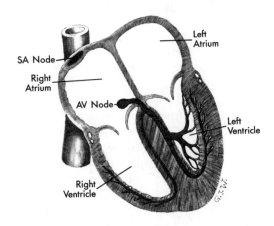

Additional Question → How might you recognize from *where* in
the heart the escape pacemaker was arising? (Feel free to refer to
page 192 in formulating your answer.)

Recognition of Escape Rhythms

Although under normal conditions the SA node serves as the principal pacemaker of the heart- there are times when the SA node may give up or falter in this function. This may occur as the result of cardiac disease (i.e., from sick sinus syndrome or infarction of the SA node)- or as a normal phenomenon (as when the rate of sinus node firing decreases during sleep, or when an individual is put under anesthesia).

If (for *whatever* reason) the SA node *fails* to initiate the electrical impulse- another (i.e., *escape*) pacemaker will hopefully assume the pacemaker function. Most often this escape focus will arise from the AV node- but it could also arise from elsewhere in one of the atria (in the form of an *atrial* escape rhythm). If neither the atria nor the AV node respond- an *idioventricular* escape rhythm (from a site in the ventricles) may assume the pacemaker function.

Intrinsic rates of AV nodal and ventricular escape pacemakers tend to follow a logical sequence. Thus, the usual **AV nodal *escape* rate** is *between* **40** and **60** beats/minute (or just *below* the limit for sinus bradycardia). The usual **idioventricular *escape* rate** is *between* **20** to **40** beats/minute (or just *below* the usual AV nodal escape rate).

As discussed on page 192- additional clues that suggest the site of the escape pacemaker are forthcoming from assessment of QRS morphology and the nature of associated atrial activity (or the *lack* thereof). As a result of their *SUPRAventricular* location- atrial and junctional escape pacemakers typically produce a QRS complex that is narrow and similar (if not identical) in appearance to the QRS complex of sinus conducted beats. In contrast- the QRS complex of ventricular escape beats is wide and very different in appearance from sinus conducted beats.

P waves regularly precede atrial escape beats. They are often (but not always) associated with junctional escape beats (as illustrated on page 143). In contrast- P waves are usually *not* associated with ventricular escape beats (although *retrograde* P waves can occasionally be seen).

Practice: *What is the rhythm?*

Use the **4 Question Approach** to interpret the rhythm shown below.

Lead II

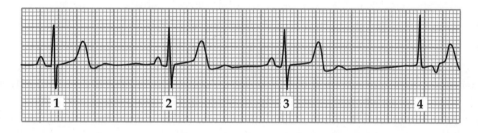

Questions:

1. Is beat #4 in the above tracing a *premature* beat- or an *escape* beat?

> HINT- Be sure to determine the *underlying* rhythm first (i.e., from assessment of beats #1, 2, and 3)- *before* answering this question.

2. From where in the heart is beat #4 likely to arise?

Interpretation:

The easiest way to interpret the rhythm that appears on page 195 is to:

1. Initially *ignore* the different looking beat (i.e., beat #4).
2. Determine the *underlying* rhythm.
3. Return to beat #4 (i.e., to the unusual looking beat).

The *overall* rhythm on page 195 is clearly *not* regular. If we initially *ignore* the different look-ing beat (i.e., beat #4)- the R-R interval for the first 3 beats *is* regular. By the **4 Question Approach**- the QRS complex for these first 3 beats is *narrow*- and each QRS is preceded by a normal appearing (i.e., *upright* in lead II) P wave. Thus, the underlying mechanism of this rhythm is *sinus*- in this case **sinus bradycardia** at a rate of just *under* 50 beats/minute (since the R-R interval between beats #1-2 and #2-3 is just *over* 6 large boxes in duration).

The *KEY* question to answer in assessing the nature of beat #4 is whether this beat occurs early or late. Since the R-R interval preceding beat #4 is clearly *longer* than the R-R interval between the sinus conducted beats- we can say that this beat occurs *later* than expected. Beat #4 is therefore an *escape* beat. Its occurrence is *fortunate*- because without this "escape" beat there may have been a much longer pause without any cardiac rhythm at all.

As discussed on pages 191-194- escape beats generally arise from one of three possible sites: 1) from the atria; 2) from the AV node; or 3) from the ventricles. The fact that the QRS complex of beat #4 is *narrow* essentially rules out a ventricular escape site. Moreover, because this QRS complex looks *different* than the QRS of sinus conducted beats- the escape focus is unlikely to be coming from the atria. This makes it most likely that the escape focus arises from the AV node- which is the most common site of origin for escape beats or rhythms. This also explains the somewhat different appearance of beat #4 (*See page 192*)- and the negative (i.e., *retrograde*) P wave that follows this escape beat (*See page 143*).

> **Note** → An *alternative* (albeit much less commonly encountered) explanation for why beat #4 is narrow may be that the escape pacemaker is arising from a point *low down* (but *still in*) the conduction system- as might occur if the site of the escape focus was *below* the AV node in the bundle of His.

Practice: *What is the rhythm?*

Use the **4 Question Approach** to interpret the rhythm shown below.

HINT- Begin by determining the *underlying* rhythm (which can be done by focusing on the initial 4 beats in this tracing). Then *one at a time*- look at *each* of the abnormal beats (i.e., beats #5, 6, 7, and 10)- to see if they occur *early* or *late.*

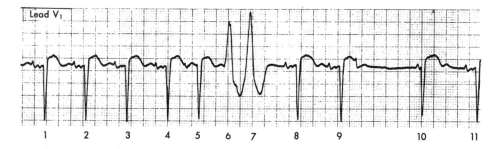

Questions:

1. Are there *premature* beats on this tracing? If so- *what type(s)* ?

2. Is there an *escape* beat? If so- *what type* ?

Interpretation:

The *KEY* to interpreting the tracing that appears on page 197 lies with first determining the *underlying* rhythm. This can be done by focusing on the initial 4 beats on the tracing. By the **4 Question Approach**- the QRS complex for these first 4 beats is *narrow*- and each QRS is preceded by a normal appearing P wave with a constant PR interval. Thus, the *underlying* mechanism of this rhythm is **sinus**.

Beat #5 occurs *earlier* than anticipated. The QRS complex of this beat is narrow and remarkably similar to the QRS complex of the sinus conducted beats. A premature P wave appears to precede beat #5- although admittedly this P wave is difficult to see because it is small in size and partially hidden by the preceding T wave (i.e., the T wave of beat #4). Premature beat #5 must therefore be a **PAC**.

Beats #6 and #7 also occur *earlier* than expected- when compared to the rate of the underlying sinus rhythm (established by the first 4 beats on the tracing). Beats #6 and #7 are both wide- very different in morphology from the normally conducted beats- and *not* preceded by premature P waves. These beats are **PVCs**- and their consecutive occurrence is termed a **ventricular couplet**. Note that this couplet is followed by a short pause- before resumption of sinus rhythm with beats #8 and #9.

Beat #10 is a *late* occurring beat. Its QRS complex looks similar- but is *not* identical to the QRS complex of sinus conducted beats (i.e., the S wave of this beat is not quite as deep as it is with the sinus conducted beats). It is the *timing* of beat #10 (i.e., its *late* occurrence)- that defines it as an *escape* beat. Although a P wave *does* precede this beat- the PR interval is far too short for the beat to be sinus conducted. This confirms the etiology of beat #10 as a **junctional escape** beat.

> **PEARL** → In clinical practice- the most common cause of a pause in a rhythm is a **blocked PAC**. This is the cause of the relative pause that occurs in this case *between* beats #9 and #10. As emphasized in the Note on page 160- it would be ever so easy to overlook the *blocked* PAC that notches the terminal portion of the T wave of beat #9- *unless* one regularly examined the T wave at the beginning of each pause- and compared the shape of this T wave (which is *notched* in this case)- to the shape of the T wave of normally conducted beats (which is *smooth* in this case).

<u>Escape Rhythms</u>: *From what site?*

- ECG Recognition -

Use the **4 Question Approach** to interpret the rhythms shown below.

Lead II

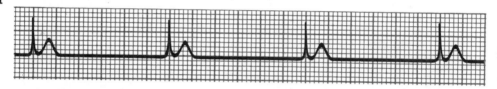

Lead II

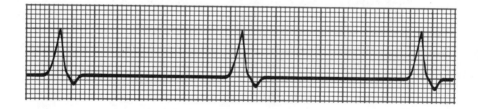

<u>**Question**</u> → From where in the heart would you expect the above rhythms to arise? (Feel free to refer to pages 192-194 in formulating your answer.)

Interpretation:

Both of the rhythms that appear on page 199 are regular. In the **TOP rhythm**- the QRS complex is narrow and not associated with any atrial activity. The R-R interval is 6 large boxes in duration- which means that the heart rate is 50 beats/minute. This is an ***AV nodal (junctional) escape* rhythm**.

In the **BOTTOM rhythm**- the QRS complex is clearly wide. No atrial activity is seen. The R-R interval is approximately 8 large boxes in duration- which corresponds to a heart rate of just under 40 beats/minute. This is an ***idioventricular escape* rhythm**.

Clinical Notes → As suggested on page 194- escape rhythms most commonly arise from a focus *within* the AV node. The usual escape rate of an AV nodal rhythm is *between* 40 to 60 beats/minute- so the rate of the junctional rhythm that appears on page 199 falls well within this range. It is important to appreciate that the presence of a junctional rhythm per se does *not* necessarily imply cardiac pathology- since otherwise healthy young adults may transiently manifest this rhythm as a *normal* phenomenon in situations that are commonly associated with sinus node slowing (i.e., during sleep or induction of anesthesia).

In contrast, the presence of an **I**dio**V**entricular **R**hythm (i.e., **IVR**) is much more likely to be associated with cardiac pathology. In particular- *slow IVR* is one of the most common bradyarrhythmias seen in the setting of cardiac arrest.

Treatment of escape rhythms will depend on the clinical condition of the patient and the setting in which the escape rhythm occurs. Thus, no treatment at all would be needed for an AV nodal escape rhythm if the patient was otherwise healthy and hemodynamically stable. On the other hand, the occurrence of a slow IVR in the setting of cardiac arrest is clear indication for treatment with either drugs (i.e.,atropine, dopamine or epinephrine)- and/or with cardiac pacing.

Ventricular Rhythms

- Escape Rhythm vs Ventricular Tachycardia -

Examine the 3 tracings that are shown below. From where in the heart would you expect each rhythm to arise?

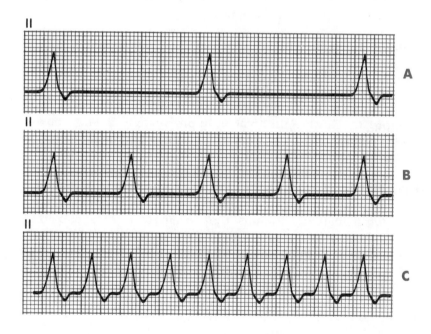

Additional Question → Are the heart rates for each of the above rhythms what you would expect?

Answer:

Each of the rhythms that appear on page 201 is regular. The QRS complex is uniformly wide- and there is no sign of atrial activity in any of the tracings. A *ventricular* etiology is therefore likely in each case:

- **Example A**- The R-R interval is 8 large boxes in duration- which corresponds to a heart rate of just *under* **40 beats/minute**. This rate falls *within* the usual range anticipated for an **idioventricular escape rhythm** in adults (i.e., *between* 20-40 beats/minute).

- **Example B**- The R-R interval is 4 large boxes in duration- which corresponds to a heart rate of **75 beats/minute**. This rate is clearly faster than what one would normally expect for an idioventricular escape pacemaker . . . (*See page 203*).

- **Example C**- The R-R interval is approximately 2 large boxes in duration- which corresponds to a heart rate of *about* **150 beats/minute**. This is **ventricular tachycardia (VT)**.

Clinical Notes ➔ With the exception of the chaotic variability of ventricular fibrillation- the sustained ventricular rhythms are most often regular (or at least *fairly* regular) rhythms that originate from a site in the ventricles. Ventricular rhythms may arise either as **escape** rhythms (if supraventricular pacemakers fail)- or as **usurping** rhythms (when the ventricular focus accelerates and *takes over* the pacemaking function from the preexisting supraventricular pacemaker).

Regarding the rhythms that appear on page 201- **Example A** illustrates the phenomenon of "escape", in which a slow IVR arises in a *rescue attempt* because higher (i.e., supraventricular) pacemakers in the SA node, atria, or AV node have either slowed down to a greater degree or have failed completely. In contrast- **Example C** illustrates the phenomenon of "usurpation", in which the ventricular focus has *accelerated* to take over the rhythm. If left untreated- VT is potentially life-threatening (because of the risk of deteriorating to ventricular fibrillation).

AIVR

- <u>A</u>ccelerated <u>I</u>dio<u>V</u>entricular <u>R</u>hythm -

Use the **4 *Question* Approach** to interpret the rhythm shown below.

<u>HINT</u>- This is one of the ventricular rhythms that was shown on page 201.

Lead II

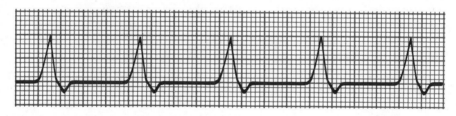

<u>Question</u> → Is the above rhythm a *slower* form of VT? or is it rather a *faster* form of an idioventricular *escape* rhythm? (Feel free to refer to page 202 in formulating your answer.)

Interpretation:

Applying the **4 Question Approach** to the rhythm that appears on page 203- we note the following:

    i) The QRS complex is clearly *wide* (i.e., *more* than *half* a large box in duration).

    ii) The rhythm is *regular.* The R-R interval is 4 large boxes in duration- which corresponds to a heart rate of **75 beats/minute**.

    iii) & iv) There are no P waves (or other signs of atrial activity).

Comment → The rhythm that appears on page 203 is commonly referred to as **AIVR** (i.e., **A**ccelerated **I**dio**V**entricular **R**hythm). The name tells all. That is- the rhythm is almost certainly of *ventricular* origin (given marked widening of the QRS complex and the absence of atrial activity)- and the ventriclar rate (of 75 beats/minute) is *"accelerated"* with respect to the usual rate of a slow IVR (which is typically between 20-40 beats/minute). *Hence the term "AIVR"* . . . .

    Instead of AIVR, some clinicians call this rhythm**"slow VT"**- so as to acknowledge that the rhythm is *faster* than a slow idioventricular rhythm- but *not* fast enough to qualify as "true VT". We feel the term AIVR is preferable because it more accurately reflects the clinical role of this arrhythmia. AIVR is most commonly seen in the settings of cardiac arrest and acute myocardial infarction- especially in the moments *just after* reperfusion of the infarct-related artery (as may occur immediately following administration of thrombolytic therapy). Surprisingly, many patients *remain* hemodynamically stable in association with AIVR (because adequate perfusion may still occur). Thus, the rhythm may serve the *lifesaving* function of "escape" in cases when supraventricular pacemakers have either slowed or failed completely. Even when AIVR arises as a "usurping" rhythm that *takes over* the pacemaking function from an otherwise adequate supraventricular pacemaker- it is usually a relatively *benign* rhythm (compared to the potentially *life-threatening* nature of VT).

Practice: *What is the rhythm?*

Use the **4 *Question Approach*** to interpret the rhythm shown below.

> HINT- Begin by determining the *underlying* rhythm- which can be done by focusing first on the *normal* appearing beats in the tracing (i.e., on beats #1, 2, 9, and 10). Then turn your attention to the run of *abnormal* beats (i.e., beats #3 through #8).

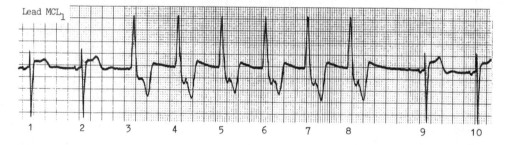

Questions:

1. Is it likely that the 6-beat run of *anomalous* (i.e., *abnormal* looking) complexes represents a "usurping" rhythm- or a rhythm of "escape" ?

2. Clinically- what will be the most important factor(s) in determining whether the above rhythm should be treated?

Interpretation:

As suggested- the easiest way to interpret the rhythm that appears on page 205 is to:

     1. Initially *ignore* the run of *anomalous* beats (i.e., beats #3 through #8).
     2. Focus first instead on the *normal* appearing beats- to try to determine the underlying rhythm.
     3. Then return to the run of abnormal looking beats.

The *normal* appearing beats in this tracing are the first two beats (#1 and 2)- and the last two beats (#9 and 10). By the **4 Question Approach**- the QRS complex for each of these normal appearing beats is *narrow*- and each QRS is preceded by a similar looking P wave with a constant PR interval. The *underlying* rhythm is therefore **sinus**.

Sinus rhythm is interrupted by the 6-beat run of anomalous complexes- beginning with beat #3. This beat is *not* premature. Instead, it is an *escape* beat that arises because of the slight slowing of the sinus pacemaker. Retrograde P waves notch the T waves of beats #4 to #8. After a short pause, sinus rhythm resumes with beat #9.

Note how QRS morphology changes dramatically with beat #3- a fact that should strongly suggest a *ventricular* etiology for this beat (as well as the run that follows). The R-R interval between beats in the run is fairly regular and just under 4 large boxes in duration- which corresponds to a rate of between 75-80 beats/minute. Thus, the run represents an episode of **AIVR**.

Clinical Notes → Two factors are most important for determining the optimal approach to management of AIVR: 1) The clinical setting in which the rhythm occurs; and 2) the patient's clinical condition and hemodynamic status. For example, given the reasonable heart rate during the run of AIVR on page 205- no treatment at all would be needed if the patient was asymptomatic and normotensive. On the other hand, an attempt to speed up the decelerating (i.e., *defaulting*) sinus pacemaker (with either atropine or pacing) would be indicated if the patient was hypotensive and/or symptomatic.

Practice: *What is the rhythm?*

Use the **4 *Question Approach*** to interpret the rhythm shown below.

HINT- There are *two* possible interpretations that may be correct !!!

Lead II

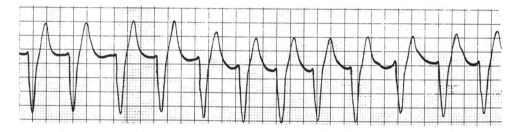

Questions:

1. Is the rhythm *completely* regular? *Are ventricular rhythms always precisely regular-* or can there be *some* variability in the ventricular rate?

2. If the etiology of the above rhythm was supraventricular- how might you explain the presence of QRS widening?

Interpretation:

Applying the **4 *Question Approach*** to the rhythm that appears on page 207- we note the following:

> i) The QRS complex is *wide* (i.e., definitely *more* than *half* a large box in duration).

> ii) Although it may *appear* on initial inspection that this rhythm is regular- *it is not* ! Careful measurement *with* **calipers** reveals that the R-R interval varies (albeit slightly) from one beat to the next.

> iii) & iv) There are no P waves (or other signs of atrial activity).

> > **Comment** → This is a difficult tracing in that one *cannot* be certain as to the true etiology of the rhythm. We feel *either* of two interpretations are *equally* correct: 1) Atrial fibrillation; or 2) AIVR.
> >
> > As noted above- the R-R interval *continually* varies (albeit slightly) from beat to beat in this tracing. This finding of an *irregularly irregular* rhythm in the absence of atrial activity suggests the diagnosis of **atrial fibrillation**- here with a *controlled* ventricular response. If this were the rhythm, QRS widening might be explained by preexisting bundle branch block.
> >
> > On the other hand- this rhythm could also represent **AIVR**. Although sustained ventricular rhythms (i.e., slow IVR, AIVR, and VT) are *usually* regular- there may at times be some variability in the ventricular response.

KEY → Do *NOT* be disturbed by the fact that two interpretations are possible for the rhythm that appears on page 207- or by the *impossibility* of determining with certainty from this single rhythm strip what the "true" rhythm is. *Many arrhythmias have more than one valid interpretation.* Instead we hope you feel satisfied if you came up with *either* of the above interpretations- and *especially* satisfied if you *considered* both of them!

Practice: *What is the rhythm?*

Use the **4 Question Approach** to interpret the rhythm shown below.

> HINT- Once again, there is *more* than one possible interpretation for this
> arrhythmia.

Lead II

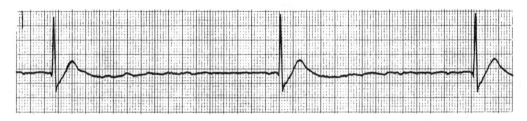

Question → From where in the heart would you expect the above
rhythm to arise?

Interpretation:

Applying the **4 *Question Approach*** to the rhythm that appears on page 209- we note the following:

i) Although the QRS complex looks to be *wide*- it is difficult to be sure if this is so from this single monitoring lead (because of the uncertain boundary between the end of the QRS complex and the beginning of the ST segment).

ii) The heart rate is exceedingly slow. Because only three QRS complexes are seen, assessment of regularity must be based on relatively limited information. What can be said is that there is slight variability in the ventricular response- and that the heart rate is in the range of about 20 beats/minute (since R-R intervals for the few beats shown are 16 and 14 large boxes, respectively).

iii) & iv) There are no P waves (or other signs of atrial activity).

Comment → The rhythm that appears on page 209 is an exceedingly slow (and at least somewhat irregular) *escape* rhythm- without evidence of associated atrial activity. Although the slow rate and QRS appearance is most consistant with a *ventricular* etiology (in the form of a **slow IVR**)- the rhythm *could* be arising from somewhere in the conduction system (either in the AV node or the bundle of His)- if the QRS complex turned out to narrow. Alternatively, the rhythm could be atrial fibrillation with an exceedingly slow ventricular response (since this rhythm *is* irregular). Clearly- a *longer* rhythm strip and/or additional monitoring leads are needed to be certain. However- *regardless* of what the true rhythm turns out to be- clinical implications and therapeutic priorities are the same- *the rate MUST be sped up* ! The treatment of choice for bradycardia of this degree is cardiac pacing- although administration of atropine and/or a pressor agent (i.e., dopamine or epinephrine) is often tried first,

---

Section 1F- *Rhythms of Cardiac Arrest*

V Fib

- *Ventricular Fibrillation* -

Interpret the rhythm shown below- obtained from a patient in cardiac arrest. Is there any evidence of *organized* electrical activity?

Lead II

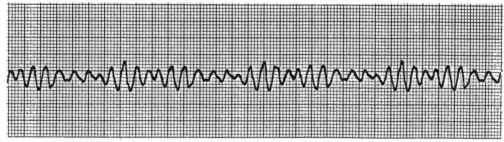

Additional Questions:

1. Clinically- what is the most important parameter to establish in association with the above rhythm? What treatment is indicated?

2. What would you suspect clinically if a patient with the above rhythm was alert and responsive?

Interpretation:

The rhythm that appears on page 211 is completely chaotic *without* any evidence of organized electrical activity. Instead, there is an irregular zig-zag pattern in which electrical waveforms continuously vary in size and shape. This is ***ventricular fibrillation (V Fib)***.

> **Clinical Notes** → V Fib is the most common inciting mechanism of cardiac arrest. As might be imagined by its totally chaotic appearance- there can be no meaningful perfusion with this rhythm. Immediate unsynchronized electrical countershock (i.e., *defibrillation*) is the treatment of choice. Because V Fib is (*by definition!*) a *non-perfusing* rhythm- the patient will die unless treatment is begun within a very short period of time (i.e., usually *within* 4-6 minutes). Administration of drugs (i.e., epinephrine)- and performance of CPR may briefly prolong the period of *potential viability.* Practically speaking, however- electrical defibrillation will virtually *always* be needed for there to be conversion of V Fib to a perfusing rhythm. The principle for the effect of this unsynchronized countershock is based on the premise that the electrical discharge will interrupt the otherwise self-sustaining process of V Fib by causing the entire mass of cardiac cells to depolarize- with the hope that this interruption will then be followed by spontaneous resumption of an *organized* (and hopefully also perfusing) supraventricular rhythm.

KEY → The most important clinical parameters to establish in association with the rhythm that appears on page 211 are *pulselessness* and *unresponsiveness.* If these are *not* present (i.e., if the patient is responsive)- *then the rhythm CAN'T be V Fib* !!! In this case, it is likely that one or more monitoring leads have become detached- a very common occurrence in the flurry of activity that is typically seen during cardiopulmonary resuscitation.

VT

- *Ventricular Tachycardia* -

Interpret the rhythm shown below- obtained from a patient in cardiac arrest. Is there evidence of *organized* electrical activity?

Lead II

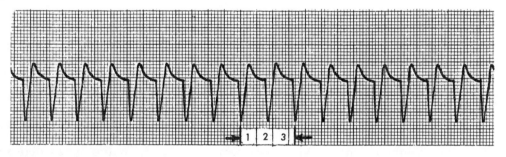

Additional Questions:

1. Clinically- what is the most important parameter to establish in association with the above rhythm?

2. What is the heart rate? Which entities should be considered in the differential diagnosis for this tachycardia?

Interpretation:

The rhythm that appears on page 213 is a regular **<u>W</u>ide-<u>C</u>omplex <u>T</u>achycardia (WCT)**- without evidence of associated atrial activity. The heart rate is approximately 170 beats/minute. Although the etiology of this rhythm *could* be supraventricular (with either aberrant conduction or preexisting bundle branch block)- **ventricular tachycardia (VT)** must be assumed until proven otherwise (*page 181*)!

That the rate is approximately 170 beats/minute can be determined by the '*Every OTHER Beat Method*' that was previously discussed (*See pages 55-58*). Selecting the QRS complex in the middle of the rhythm strip as our starting point (because the S wave of this complex falls right on a heavy grid line)- it can be seen that the R-R interval for *every other beat* (i.e., *half* the rate)- is between 3 and 4 large boxes in duration. Thus *half* the rate is about 85 beats/minute- and the actual rate = 85 X 2 = **170 beats/minute**.

<u>**Clinical Notes**</u> ➔ In contrast to V Fib- VT is *not* necessarily a non-perfusing rhythm. Because VT is an *organized* arrhythmia, meaningful cardiac contraction may sometimes occur- so that some patients may remain awake, alert and hemodynamically stable *despite* persistence of VT for surprisingly *long* periods of time (i.e., of minutes, hours- *and even days!*). As a result, the first priority when assessing *any* patient with a WCT of uncertain etiology should be to determine whether that patient is hemodynamically stable. If not- immediate electrical cardioversion will be in order. On the other hand, if the patient *IS* alert, normotensive and relatively asymptomatic- then medical therapy (i.e., usually with lidocaine or procainamide) is a reasonable initial approach- with the precaution of remaining *ever ready* to immediately cardiovert the patient should hemodynamic decompensation occur at *any* time during the treatment process.

Asystole

Interpret the rhythm shown below- obtained from a patient in cardiac arrest. Is there any evidence of electrical activity?

Lead II

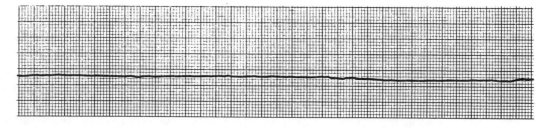

Additional Questions:

1. Clinically- what is the most important parameter to establish in association with the above rhythm? What treatment is indicated?

2. Can you think of anything *other than* asystole that might produce a flat-line recording in a single monitoring lead?

Interpretation:

A *flat-line* recording is seen in the tracing that appears on page 215. This is **asystole**. The term *asystole* literally means "no systole"- which translates to the complete absence of mechanical *and* electrical activity. Treatment consists of performance of CPR (since by definition- asystole is a *non-perfusing* rhythm)- administration of medication (especially epinephrine and atropine)- and application of cardiac pacing. Unfortunately, regardless of whatever interventions are tried- the prognosis for most patients with asystole will be exceedingly poor.

Clinical Notes → On rare occasions, V Fib may "masquerade" as asystole. Like any other electrocardiographic complex, the undulations of V Fib possess a predominant vector of electrical activity. Should this vector be oriented *perpendicular* to the electrical axis of the monitor lead being recorded- a flat line will be observed in that particular lead. Fortunately, this phenomenon can be *easily* recognized- simply by monitoring the patient in *more* than a single lead. This is important clinically because V Fib should be treated with defibrillation- whereas shocking asystole may make the rhythm even more resistant to treatment than it already is.

As is the case for other rhythms that occur in association with cardiac arrest- the most important clinical parameters to establish when confronted with a flat line recording are that the patient *truly* is pulseless and unresponsive. In addition to the phenomenon of fine V Fib masquerading as asystole (described above)- other conditions that may spuriously produce a flat line recording on the monitor screen *despite* the presence of electrical and mechanical activity include a malfunctioning monitor, inadvertent turning down of the monitor amplitude gain, and loose or detached monitoring leads. Practically speaking- these technical errors are all much more common causes of a flat-line recording than the rare phenomenon of V Fib masquerading as asystole.

Bradycardia/PEA

- *P*ulseless *E*lectrical *A*ctivity -

Interpret the rhythm shown below- obtained from a patient in cardiac arrest.

Lead II

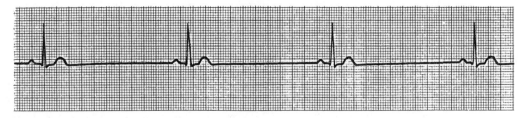

Questions:

1. What is the mechanism of the above rhythm? What is the heart rate?

2. How would you interpret the above rhythm if told that it was obtained from a patient who did *not* have a pulse?

Interpretation:

The rhythm that appears on page 217 is exceedingly slow. Nevertheless, the rhythm is regular. With an R-R interval of just under 12 large boxes in duration, we estimate the heart rate to be approximately **25 beats/minute** (i.e., 300 ÷ 12).

Despite the slow rate- the QRS complex is narrow- and each QRS is preceded by a normal appearing (i.e., *upright* in lead II) P wave with a constant and normal PR interval. Thus the *mechanism* of the rhythm is *sinus*- and the rhythm is **sinus bradycardia**.

Clinical Notes → Our interpretation of the rhythm that appears on page 217 would change dramatically if we were told that the patient did *not* have a pulse. In this case we would describe the condition as either **EMD** or **PEA** (i.e., **E**lectro**M**echanical **D**issociation- or **P**ulseless **E**lectrical **A**ctivity)- depending on the terminology one chose to employ. Both terms acknowledge the presence of electrical activity on the monitor (in the form of an *organized* ECG rhythm)- but in the *absence* of effective mechanical contraction (i.e., *there is NO pulse!*). PEA rhythms (including EMD) most often arise as the electrical manifestation of some other underlying disorder or clinical catastrophe (i.e., rupture of a ventricular or aortic aneurysm, massive pulmonary embolus, tension pneumothorax, pericardial tamponade, severe hypovolemia, etc.). Practically speaking- realistic chances for meaningful survival (i.e., with intact neurologic function) depend on *prompt* discovery and *correction* of the underlying cause of PEA/EMD (which unfortunately will *not* be possible in many cases). Additional treatment measures include performance of CPR (since *by definition* PEA is a *non-perfusing* rhythm)- and administration of epinephrine (in the hope of improving coronary perfusion).

Slow IVR

- Slow IdioVentricular Rhythm -

Interpret the rhythm shown below- obtained from a patient in cardiac arrest.

Lead II

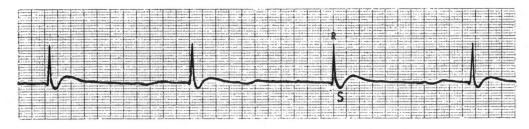

Questions:

1. How does the mechanism of the above rhythm differ from the mechanism of the rhythm shown on page 217?

2. From where in the heart would you expect the above rhythm to arise?

Interpretation:

The rhythm that appears on page 219 is regular and slow. However, in contrast to the rhythm that appears on page 217- the mechanism in this case is *not* sinus (because atrial activity is absent).

The rate of the rhythm on page 219 is just *under* 30 beats/minute (since the R-R interval is about 11 large boxes in duration). However, it is difficult to be certain from where in the heart the rhythm arises. If one includes the wide S wave in measurement of QRS duration, there is no question that the QRS is prolonged. If this were the case, then this would be a **slow idioventricular escape rhythm** (*See also pages 199-202*).

On the other hand- the component labeled S could be the beginning of the ST segment rather than the terminal portion of the QRS complex. In this case, the QRS complex would *not* be prolonged- which would suggest that this escape rhythm was arising from somewhere *within* the conduction system (i.e., either from the AV node despite the slow rate- or from lower down in the bundle of His).

Clinical Notes → Practically speaking- clinical and therapeutic implications of this rhythm will be the same *regardless* of whether or not the QRS complex is wide (and *regardless* of from where in the heart the rhythm is arising). In either case- the bottom line clinical need is that the rate of this rhythm *must* be sped up!

<u>Agonal Rhythm</u>

Interpret the rhythm shown below- obtained from a patient in cardiac arrest. Is there evidence of *organized* electrical activity?

Lead II

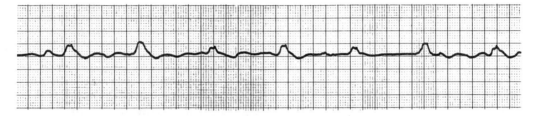

<u>Questions:</u>

1. How does the mechanism of the above rhythm differ from the mechanism of the rhythm shown on page 219 ?

2. Would you imagine that the above rhythm will be associated with effective cardiac contraction?

Interpretation:

Although at first glance the rhythm that appears on page 221 may seem to resemble a slow IVR- this is *not* the mechanism that is operative. Instead, it can be seen that the complexes in this rhythm are exceedingly wide (i.e., *more* than 0.20 second in duration!)- and totally amorphous. There is no sign of atrial activity. This is an **agonal rhythm.** In contrast, the QRS complexes that appear on page 219 are all uniform in morphology- which implies the presence of an *organized* (albeit markedly slowed) rhythm.

> **Clinical Notes** → In general, *agonal* rhythm (as its name implies) is a manifestation of a *dying* heart. Surprisingly, the sporadic electrical activity associated with an agonal rhythm may continue for minutes (and sometimes even hours) after meaningful cardiac function has ceased. Isolated and grouped idioventricular complexes (or the amorphous waveforms seen on page 221) may appear- be interrupted by long periods of asystole- and then reappear on the monitor. Clinically, the significance of an agonal rhythm (as well as its treatment) is similar to that of asystole (as discussed on pages 215-216).

Practice: *What is the rhythm?*

Use the **4 *Question Approach*** to interpret the rhythm shown below.

> <u>HINT</u>- Determine the underlying rhythm first (i.e., by assessing the initial 3 beats on this tracing). Then assess beat #4- and finally address what happens following beat #5.

Lead II

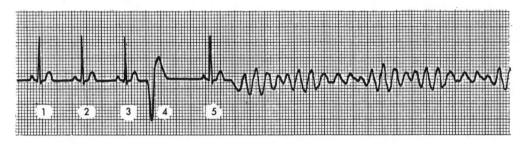

Interpretation:

The initial *underlying* mechanism for the rhythm that appears on page 223 is **sinus tachycardia**- as evidenced by the first 3 beats on the tracing. The QRS complex for these beats is narrow- and each QRS is preceded by a normal appearing (i.e., *upright* in lead II) P wave with a normal and constant PR interval. The R-R interval is just under 3 large boxes in duration- which corresponds to a heart rate of 105 beats/minute.

Beat #4 occurs early. This premature beat is wide and not associated with atrial activity. Beat #4 is a **PVC**.

Sinus rhythm resumes momentarily with beat #5- and is then interrupted by the sudden onset of **ventricular fibrillation (V Fib)**.

> **Clinical Notes** → In the setting of cardiac arrest, the occurrence of ventricular ectopy (i.e., PVCs) is worrisome because of the risk that a PVC may occur at a *vulnerable* point in the cardiac cycle and precipitate deterioration of the rhythm to V Fib.

<u>Practice</u>: *What is the rhythm?*

Use the **4 *Question* Approach** to interpret the rhythm shown below.

> <u>HINT</u>- Sequentially analyze the 3 different rhythms that are shown in the tracing below.

Lead II

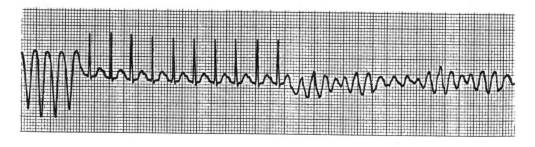

Interpretation:

The rhythm that appears on page 225 begins (for the first 4 beats) with what appears to be ***ventricular tachycardia (VT)*** at an extremely rapid rate. This is followed by a 10-beat run of an **SVT** (i.e., narrow QRS complex- or *SUPRAventricular* tachycardia) at a rate of about 210 beats/minute- which then deteriorates to ***ventricular fibrillation (V Fib)***.

> **Clinical Notes** → Although it is difficult to be certain of the etiology of the supraventricular rhythm that appears in the middle of the tracing on page 225- the rapidity of its rate (i.e., 210 beats/minute) and the absence of atrial activity are most consistent with PSVT (*See pages 125-128*).

Artifact

Interpret the rhythm shown below- obtained from a patient in cardiac arrest. The patient has just been defibrillated.

> HINT- A faint but *definite* pulse was palpated at the time this tracing was recorded.

Lead II

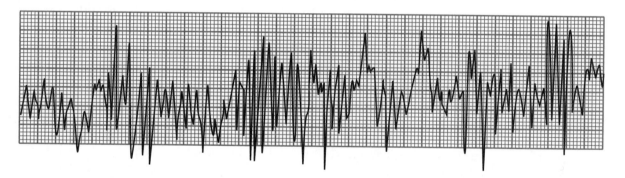

Additional Questions:

1. Should this patient be defibrillated a second time?

2. In view of the hint provided above- what do you suspect has happened?

Interpretation:

The rhythm that appears on page 227 is comprised of a bizarre series of vertical lines occurring at an extremely rapid rate. This rhythm is incompatible with the physical finding of a palpable pulse- and should make you strongly suspect the presence of **artifact**.

The patient should *not* be defibrillated. Instead, an attempt should be made to determine the cause of the artifact and to try to correct the problem- so as to be able to determine the patient's *true* rhythm.

Clinical Notes → Artifactual rhythms are very commonly seen during cardiopulmonary resuscitation. This should not be unexpected considering the usual scenario in which a large number of health care providers are feverishly working at the bedside in a concerted effort to save the patient. Awareness of potential *artifact-generating* tasks often goes a long way toward assisting in the recognition of artifactual rhythms. Thus, artifact may be caused by performance of CPR, intubation, ventilation, defibrillation, intravenous cannulation, and drawing of arterial blood gases. In addition, monitor leads often become loose or are knocked off completely during resuscitative efforts. For all of these reasons- one should *always* check for the presence of a pulse and patient responsiveness *before* proceding with defibrillation of a rhythm that superficially resembles V Fib (such as the tracing that appears on the preceding page). If the patient responds or a pulse is palpated- *then the rhythm is not V Fib* !

PEARL → Return for a moment to the example of V Fib that appears on the front of page 211. Note how that tracing differs from the picture shown on page 227- in that artifactual waveforms are of much greater amplitude and are clearly more vertically oriented than the waveforms associated with V Fib. These two clues (i.e., increased waveform amplitude and geometrically vertical orientation) are strongly suggestive of the presence of artifact.

<u>Practice</u>: *What is the rhythm?*

Interpret the rhythm strips shown below- obtained in succession from a patient in cardiac arrest. The *arrows* in each case indicate the point at which an electrical discharge was delivered to the patient.

Lead II

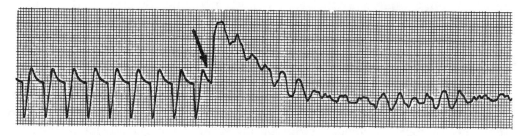

Lead II

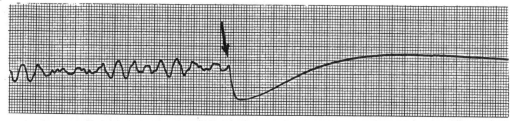

<u>Question</u> → What type of electrical discharge (i.e., synchronized or unsynchronized shock) would be indicated in each case? *Describe what happened.*

Interpretation:

The rhythm shown in the <u>Top Tracing</u> on page 229 begins as a 9-beat run of VT (at a rate of approximately 180 beats/minute). Because VT is an *organized* electrical rhythm (with a reentry mechanism)- it often responds to *synchronized* cardioversion (i.e., to delivery of an electrical discharge synchronized to the *least* vulnerable point in the cardiac cycle). Unfortunately in this case- cardioversion precipitates deterioration of the rhythm to V Fib.

The <u>Bottom Tracing</u> on page 229 begins as V Fib. Because V Fib is a completely chaotic and *disorganized* rhythm- synchronized cardioversion can *not* be used (i.e., there is no organized QRS complex to "synch" to). Treatment of V Fib should be with *unsynchronized* countershock- which unfortunately in this case results in further deterioration of the rhythm to asystole.

Mechanisms of Cardiac Arrest:

The three major *mechanisms* of cardiac arrest are shown on page 229: 1) V Fib; 2) VT; and 3) bradycardia-asystole. We have already noted on page 212 how **V Fib** is the most commonly encountered mechanism (i.e., *initial* rhythm) of cardiac arrest- especially for episodes that occur *outside* of the hospital setting. It is far less common for emergency rescuers to encounter a patient with out-of-hospital cardiac arrest in **ventricular tachycardia** *(pages 213-214)*- although it may be that VT had *initially* been present in some (if not many) cases of out-of-hospital cardiac arrest- and had *already deteriorated* to V Fib by the time emergency rescuers arrived on the scene. This may explain the surprisingly frequent observation of VT as a precipitating (i.e. *initial*) mechanism of cardiac arrest that occurs *within* a hospital setting (where the period of time until trained rescuers arrive is usually much shorter).

The major remaining mechanism of cardiac arrest is comprised of rhythms included within the classification of **bradycardia-asystole**. It is estimated that this mechanism accounts for up to one third of all cases of cardiopulmonary arrest that occur *outside* of the hospital setting. Among the entities included within this group of cardiac arrest rhythms are **asystole** (page 215)- **PEA rhythms** (page 217)- and other *bradyarrhythmias*, of which **slow IVR** is probably the most common form (page 219).

Practice: *What is the rhythm?*

Interpret the rhythm shown below- obtained from a patient in cardiac arrest.

Lead II

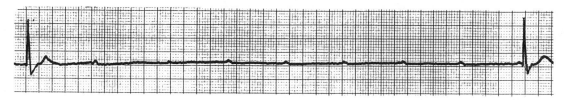

Questions:

1. Is there evidence of organized *ventricular* activity? of organized *atrial* activity?

2. How long is the pause in the above rhythm? How should this rhythm be treated?

Interpretation:

As might be imagined, the prognosis of a patient in cardiac arrest with the rhythm shown on page 231 will not be good. Organized ventricular activity *is* present- in the form of relatively normal appearing (and *not* markedly widened- if widened at all) QRS complexes that begin and end the rhythm strip. In between is a long period of **ventricular standstill**- that lasts for *more* than **7 seconds** (i.e., 38 small boxes in duration- or ≈7.6 seconds!).

Despite the lack of ventricular escape activity during the pause- *atrial* activity (in the form of slightly irregular but continually occurring P waves) are seen throughout the recording.

Clinical Notes → Realistic chances for survival with the rhythm shown on page 231 are slim. Recommendations for treatment are similar to those for other rhythms included within the classification of *bradycardia-asystole* mechanisms of cardiac arrest:

1. Performance of CPR (since perfusion is clearly inadequate).
2. Administration of medication (especially epinephrine and atropine).
3. Application of cardiac pacing (in an attempt to achieve ventricular capture- with the hope of speeding up the rate).

Pearl → Overall Perspective on Cardiac Arrest Rhythms

ECG rhythms that occur during cardiac arrest often do *not* "obey the rules." This is as might be expected given the clinical situation of a "dying heart." As a result, much more important than trying to define the specific nature of rhythms such as the one shown on page 231- is appreciation of the presence of a life-threatening bradyarrhythmia that needs to be sped up.

<u>CPR Rhythm</u>

Interpret the rhythm shown below- obtained from a patient in cardiac arrest.

   <u>HINT</u>- Full cardiopulmonary resuscitation is in progress.

Lead II

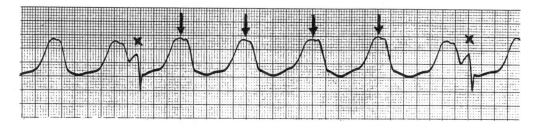

Questions:

1. What do you suspect is producing the waveforms highlighted by *arrows* in the above tracing? How could you *verify* this suspicion?

2. What do you suspect is the *underlying* rhythm?

   <u>HINT</u>- Focus on the complexes labeled " **X** ".

3. How should this patient be treated?

Interpretation:

The tracing that appears on page 233 is comprised of a number of extremely broad wave-forms (*arrows*)- that are seen to separate rare *idioventricular* escape complexes (labeled " **X** " in the tracing). The broad waveforms are too wide and amorphous to even represent an agonal rhythm (such as that shown on page 221). In view of the fact that full resuscitative efforts were in progress at the time the tracing was recorded- these broad waveforms most likely represent a *"CPR rhythm"*- in which the broad deflections result from depression of the victim's chest during each external chest compression. This suspicion can *easily* be verified- simply by ask-ing the rescue team to *stop CPR*- which should result in immediate elimination of the broad waveforms.

Given that the only evidence of spontaneous electrical activity is in the form of rare and widened idioventricular beats- the *underlying* rhythm in this tracing is either an exceedingly slow IVR- or more likely an *agonal* rhythm.

Clinical Notes → Recommended treatment for the rhythm shown on page 233 is similar to that for the other entities included within the group of cardiac arrest rhythms known as *bradycardia-asystole* :

1. Performance of CPR (since perfusion is clearly inadequate).
2. Administration of medication (especially epinephrine and atropine).
3. Application of cardiac pacing (in an attempt to achieve ventricu-lar capture- and hopefully speed up the rate).

PEARL *(Beyond the Core)* → Note in this case that the *rate* of CPR should be increased! That is, each arrow in the tracing on page 233 has an R-R interval of about 5 large boxes in duration- which corresponds to a rate of 1 compression per second (or 60 compressions per minute)- which is significantly *slower* than the rec-ommended rate of 80-100 external chest compressions per minute!

Section 1G- AV Blocks- *Basic Concepts*

AV Blocks

- Traditional Classification -

    Diagnosis of the AV blocks is a common source of confusion for the emergency care provider not accustomed to dealing with these rhythm disturbances on a daily basis. Confusion begins with terminology, encompasses diagnosis, and extends into prognostic implications and therapeutic decision making.

> **Note** → Diagnosis of the various AV blocks need *not* be difficult! The *KEY* is to keep in mind the basic classification of the AV blocks- and to *systematically* apply the **4 *Question Approach*** to interpretation in the *same way* you apply it to evaluating any other cardiac arrhythmia.

Questions to Further Understanding:

    1. How are AV blocks traditionally classified ?

        HINT- There are *three degrees* of AV block.

Traditional Classification of the AV Blocks:

- *1° AV Block*

- *2° AV Block* :
    - Mobitz type I (= Wenckebach)
    - Mobitz type II

- *3° (= Complete) AV Block*

KEY to Understanding the Traditional Classification

- **First degree (1°) AV block**- entails conduction of *all* atrial impulses to the ventricles- but with *delay* in the process of conduction. Since all atrial impulses *are* conducted- each QRS will be preceded by a P wave and *related* to that P wave by a constant PR interval. It's just that this PR interval will be prolonged.

- **Third degree (3°) AV block**- entails a *complete block* in AV conduction- so that *none* of the atrial impulses are conducted to the ventricles. As a result, there is *no relation* between P waves and QRS complexes on the tracing. The PR interval that precedes each QRS complex will therefore *continually* change (since P waves are *unrelated* to QRS complexes).

- **Second degree (2°) AV block**- differs from 1° and 3° AV block in that there is a *partial block* in AV conduction. As a result, *some* atrial impulses are conducted to the ventricles- *but others are not*. Electrocardiographically- *some* P waves will be related to QRS complexes (because they are being conducted)- *but others will not*.

AV Blocks

- *Drawbacks of Traditional Classification* -

Questions to Further Understanding:

1. Can you think of potential *drawbacks* to the traditional classification system described on page 236? Consider the following three questions in formulating your answer:

   HINT #1- Does the degree of AV block *reliably* indicate severity of the underlying conduction disturbance? (i.e., Will 3° AV block always be *"worse"* than 1° or 2° AV block?)

   HINT #2- Where does *AV dissociation* fit into the traditional system?

   HINT #3- Does the system take into account *clinical* assessment of the patient ?

Drawbacks of Traditional Classification

There are a number of drawbacks to the traditional system for classification of the AV blocks. They include:

1. Tacit assumption that the *degree* of AV block reliably indicates the severity of the conduction disturbance (i.e., that 1° AV block is the *mildest* disorder- and that 3° AV block is necessarily the most severe).

2. Failure to account for a number of **"unclaimed terms"** that often serve as a source of confusion (i.e., AV dissociation, high grade or high degree block).

3. Failure to consider *clinical assessment* of the patient (i.e., pulse, BP, and the presence or absence of symptoms) in the evaluation process.

Consider the following two clinical vignettes:

- **Patient A-** has "only" 1° AV block- but with marked bradycardia (say, a heart rate of 20 beats/minute), resultant hypotension, and severe chest pain.

- **Patient B-** has *complete* (= 3°) AV block- but with an AV nodal escape pacemaker at a reasonable rate (say, of 50 beats/minute)- so that the patient is asymptomatic and able to maintain a normal BP = 120/80 mm Hg.

Which patient is better off? - Patient A who has "only" 1° AV block (but a heart rate of 20 beats/minute)- or Patient B with the "more severe" 3° AV block ?

> **KEY** → Much more important than the "degree" of AV block per se is the patient's *clinical condition* and *hemodynamic* status (which is why we include this information *whenever* possible as part of our interpretation).

AV Blocks

- Simplified Approach to Diagnosis -

In acknowledgement of the potential drawbacks of traditional classification, we suggest the following *simplified* approach for evaluation of the AV blocks. It entails:

1. Routine use of the **4 Question Approach** to interpretation- as for any other cardiac arrhythmia.

2. Inclusion (whenever possible) of **Clinical Assessment** in your interpretation (i.e., consideration of the pulse, BP, and the presence or absence of symptoms *in association* with the arrhythmia).

3. Use of the **KISS Method** to assist in determining the *degree* of AV block.

4. Awareness and understanding of the **"Unclaimed Terms"** (that we noted on page 238).

Simplified Approach to Diagnosis of AV Blocks

- Routine use of the **4 Question Approach**- is the easiest way to interpret an arrhythmia that might represent a type of AV block. As discussed in detail on pages 61-86- the questions entail:

    1. *Looking for* **P waves**.
    2. *Assessing for* **regularity** *of the rhythm*- with specific attention directed *not only* to the pattern of QRS complexes- but *also* to regularity (or the lack thereof) for the occurrence of P waves.
    3. *Determining* **QRS width**.
    4. *Identifying the* **relationship** *(if any) between P waves and the QRS*. Practically speaking- this is the *KEY* determinant of the nature of the AV conduction disturbance.

- Inclusion of **Clinical Assessment**- *whenever* possible. For example, failure to include the rate (of 20 beats/minute) in your interpretation of the rhythm for **Patient A** (on page 238)- *as well as* the fact that this patient was hypotensive and complaining of severe chest pain would *not* have conveyed the true clinical picture.

- Use of the **KISS** *(=* **K**eep **I**t **S**imple*) Method* - to assist in determining the *degree* of AV block. The *KISS Method* is based on the fact that *both* 1° and 3° AV blocks are usually *easy* to diagnose. Therefore- if you *know* that AV block is present, but are sure that the block is *neither* 1° nor 3°- *then the conduction disturbance MUST be a type of* 2° *AV block* !!!!

- Awareness and understanding of the **"Unclaimed" Terms**- which may serve as a source of confusion. In addition to clarifying the meaning of terms such as **high grade** and **high degree** AV block- we emphasize the importance of recognizing that 3° AV block is *not* the same as **AV dissociation**.

1° AV Block

Use the **4 *Question Approach*** to interpret the rhythm shown below.

Lead II

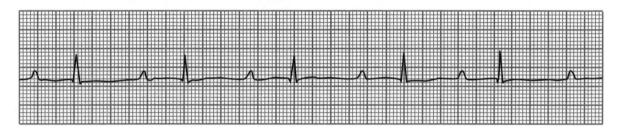

Questions:

1. Are P waves in the above tracing *related* (i.e., "married") to their respective QRS complex?

2. Is treatment indicated for this rhythm?

Interpretation:

Applying the *4 Question Approach* to the rhythm that appears on page 241- we note the following:

> i) The *width* of the QRS complex is at the upper limit of normal. That is, the QRS is about *half* a large box (or 0.10 second) in duration.

> ii) The rhythm is fairly *regular.* The R-R interval is about 6 large boxes in duration- which corresponds to a heart rate of about **50 beats/minute**.

> iii) & iv) Normal sinus (i.e., *upright* in lead II) P waves are seen throughout the tracing. Each QRS complex is *related* (i.e., "married") to its preceding P wave- as evidenced by a *fixed* PR interval (that in this case is markedly *prolonged* to about 0.44 second in duration).

> **Comment** → The rhythm on page 241 is **sinus bradycardia** at a rate of 50 beats/ minute. There is **1° AV block**.

Clinical Notes → First degree AV block is defined as a sinus rhythm in which the PR interval is prolonged to ≥**0.21 second** in duration. Since one large box on ECG grid paper corresponds to a time interval of 0.20 second- the PR interval must **clearly** be *more* **than a large box** in duration before we can say there is 1° AV block.

By itself, the finding of 1° AV block is rarely of clinical significance (and therefore does *not* require treatment). In view of its generally benign implications- and because a PR interval of 0.20-0.21 second is probably normal for many older individuals- we generally prefer *not* to diagnose 1° AV block unless the PR interval is *definitely* prolonged (i.e., to *at least* 0.22 second).

3° AV Block

- *Complete AV Block* -

Use the **4 *Question Approach*** to interpret the rhythm shown below.

> <u>HINT</u>- When assessing *regularity*- be sure to look *not only* at the ventricular rhythm- but *also* at the atrial rhythm.

Lead MCL₁

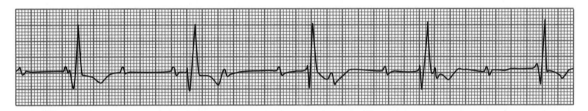

Questions:

1. Are P waves in the above tracing *related* (i.e., "married") to neighboring QRS complexes?

2. Do any of the P waves have a *chance* to conduct? That is- do at least *some* P waves occur at a point in the cardiac cycle when you would not expect the ventricles to still be in a *refractory* state (*See pages 159-160*) ?

Interpretation:

Applying the **4 Question Approach** to the rhythm that appears on page 243- we note the following:

i) The QRS complex is *wide* (i.e., clearly *more* than *half* a large box in duration).

ii) & iii) P waves are present and fairly regular. The P-P interval is between 3 and 4 large boxes in duration (which corresponds to an *atrial* rate of between 85-90 beats/minute). The *ventricular* rate is almost precisely regular- with an R-R interval of 7.5 large boxes (which corresponds to a ventricular rate of about 40 beats/minute).

iv) P waves are completely *unrelated* to neighboring QRS complexes (i.e., there is complete AV dissociation).

Comment → This is **3° (complete) AV block**- here with an atrial rate of between 85-90 beats/minute, and a ventricular rate of 40 beats/minute.

Clinical Notes → Complete AV block is said to be present when *none* of the atrial impulses are conducted to the ventricles. As a result- both the atria and ventricles will tend to discharge at their own inherent rate (which is why both atrial and ventricular rates tend to be *regular* when there is 3° AV block). P waves may precede some QRS complexes with 3° AV block, but by definition- *all* P waves are completely *unrelated* to neighboring QRS complexes (as evidenced by the fact that the PR interval *continually* changes).

The *lack* of association between atrial and ventricular activity is known as **AV dissociation**. AV dissociation may be short-lived (lasting for only a few beats)- or it may be complete, as it is with 3° AV block (in which case *none* of the P waves on the tracing will be related in any way to QRS complexes).

3° AV Block

- *Criteria for Diagnosis-*

Reexamine the tracing below (that was just presented on page 243). Note that we have numbered the QRS complexes and labeled the P waves. Using this tracing as an example- list the criteria used to make the diagnosis of 3° (complete) AV block.

HINT- Feel free to refer to page 244 in formulating your answer.

Lead MCL₁

Lead MCL$_1$

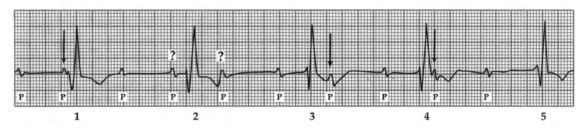

Additional Questions → Would you expect those P waves in the above tracing that are marked by arrows to conduct? Would you expect *other* P waves in the tracing to conduct?

Criteria for Diagnosis of 3° (Complete) AV Block

As noted on page 244- the condition of 3° (complete) AV block is said to be present when *none* of the atrial impulses are conducted to the ventricles. When this occurs the atria and ventricles beat *independently* at their own inherent rate. With **3° AV block** then, one *expects* to see:

1. A *regular* (or at least almost regular) atrial rate- as evidenced by a relatively *constant* P-P interval.

2. A *regular* (or at least almost regular) ventricular rate- as evidenced by a relatively *constant* R-R interval.

3. *No relationship between the two* (i.e., **complete AV dissociation**).

It should be emphasized that to be *truly* certain that 3° AV block is present there must be complete *failure* of conduction (i.e., complete AV dissociation)- ***despite adequate opportunity for normal conduction to occur.*** For example, in the tracing that appears on page 245- one would clearly *not* expect the P waves marked by arrows to conduct because the PR interval is either *too short* (as it is for the P wave that precedes beat #1)- or the P wave occurs so soon after the QRS complex that it almost certainly falls within the absolute refractory period (as it does for the P waves that immediately follow beats #3 and #4).

Admittedly, it is difficult to know if the P waves that precede and follow beat #2 (each marked by a **?**) might be able to conduct. However, it would certainly seem that most other P waves on this tracing should be occurring at points in the cardiac cycle when the ventricles should *not* be refractory.

> **Note** → The atrial rate in the tracing that appears page 245 is *not* completely regular. Occasionally in the setting of AV block or AV dissociation with a slow escape rhythm- the atrial rate will vary slightly (***ventriculophasic* sinus arrhythmia**). The mechanism for this phenomenom is *not* completely clear.

3° AV Block

- *The Level of the Block/Clinical Implications* -

We have already alluded to the fact that 3° (complete) AV block may occur at two levels: 1) **At** the level of the AV node; or 2) **Below** the AV node.

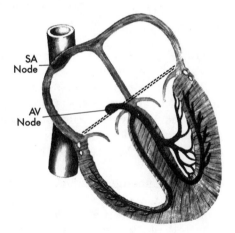

Questions:

1. What would you expect the escape pacemaker to look like if the level of 3° AV block was *at* the AV node? What if it were *below* the AV node (i.e., *below* the double dotted line in the above Figure)?

    <u>HINT</u>- Feel free to refer to pages 192-194 in formulating your answers.

2. What is the probable level of block for the tracing shown on page 245 ?

Determining the Level of 3° AV Block

- *If the level of 3° AV block is* **AT** *the AV node-* then an AV nodal rhythm should take over. The QRS of the escape pacemaker will be **narrow**, very similar (or identical) in morphology to the QRS of normally conducted beats, and occurring at a rate of between **40-60 beats/minute**. Clinically, this type of 3° AV block is most often seen in association with acute *inferior* infarction. Because the rate of the escape pacemaker is between 40-60 beats/minute, many patients remain hemodynamically stable- and do *not* require pacing despite being in complete AV block. If treatment is needed, atropine is often effective. This type of 3° AV block will often resolve spontaneously.

- *If the level of 3° AV block is* **BELOW** *the AV node-* an *idioventricular* escape pacemaker should take over. This should produce a QRS complex that is **wide**, very different in morphology from the sinus conducted beats, and occurring at a much slower rate (usually between **20-40 beats/minute**). Clinically, this type of 3° AV block is most likely to occur in association with acute *anterior* infarction. Because the level of block is much *lower* down in the conduction system- the escape pacemaker is significantly slower and much less reliable than it is for complete AV block that occurs at the level of the AV node. As a result, atropine is much less likely to be effective, and cardiac pacing will almost always be needed.

> **Note** → Exceptions clearly exist to the generalities stated above for determining the level of the AV block. For example, the QRS complex could be *wide* despite the occurrence of an AV nodal escape rhythm if the patient had preexisting bundle branch block. Alternatively, the QRS complex could be *narrow* despite arising from a lower escape pacemaker- if the escape rhythm originated from a site that was still *within* the conduction system (as might be seen with an escape focus arising from the bundle of His- *See the Note on page 196*).
>
> Regarding the rhythm that appears on page 245- one should suspect that the level of this 3° AV block is low (i.e., *below* the AV node) because the QRS complex is wide and the heart rate is *slow* (about 40 beats/minute).

3° AV Block

- *Modified Criteria for Diagnosis* -

Diagnosis of 3° AV block is often a source of confusion. Slight *modification* of the criteria presented on page 246- and addition of a fourth criterion can greatly facilitate the diagnostic process.

Modified Criteria for Diagnosis of 3° AV Block

1. A **regular** (or at least *almost* regular) atrial rate- *unless* there is marked sinus arrhythmia.
2. A **regular** (or at least *almost* regular) ventricular rate.
3. Complete AV dissociation- **despite adequate opportunity** *for normal conduction to occur.*
4. A sufficiently **slow** ventricular rate (*usually* ≤**45 beats/minute**)- to ensure adequate opportunity for normal conduction to occur.

Additional Questions:

1. Why is the ventricular response most often *regular* when there is 3° AV block?

2. What degree of AV block should you suspect is present when the ventricular response is *not* regular?

Modified Criteria for Diagnosis of 3° AV Block

1. A **regular** atrial rate (*unless* there is underlying sinus arrhythmia).
2. A **regular** (or at least *almost* regular) ventricular rate.
3. Complete AV dissociation- **despite adequate opportunity** *for normal conduction to occur.*
4. A sufficiently **slow** ventricular rate (*usually* ≤**45 beats/minute**)- to ensure adequate opportunity for normal conduction to occur.

The *KEY* to diagnosis lies with awareness of the fact that *most* of the time- **the ventricular response will be regular with 3° AV block**. This is because *none* of the supraventricular (sinus) implulses will be conducted to the ventricles if the block is complete- and *most* of the time escape rhythms (be they junctional or idioventricular) are at least fairly regular.

> If AV block is present but the ventricular response is clearly *not* regular- *then the conduction disturbance is likely to be something other than 3° AV block* (i.e., a more complicated form of 2° AV block in which there may be *transient* AV dissociation, escape beats, and the like) !!!

The reason the atrial rate will usually be regular (or at least *almost* regular) with 3° AV block is that the SA node most often continues to discharge at its usual rate. It's just that *none* of the atrial impulses are conducted to the ventricles. This results in *complete* AV dissociation (with P waves "marching through" the QRS).

As emphasized on page 246- in order to *prove* that no atrial impulses are being conducted to the ventricles, one must demonstrate that <u>*despite*</u> being given ample opportunity to conduct- P waves *don't* conduct. To do this the ventricular rate should be **slow** enough (and the rhythm strip *long* enough) to show P waves occurring at virtually *all* points in the cardiac cycle (so as to ensure *maximal opportunity* for conduction to occur). *Usually this requires a ventricular rate of **45 beats/minute** or less.* Failure of conduction is suggested by continued *regularity* of the ventricular response. Clinically- the advantage of adding this rate criterion is that it helps prevent the all too common error of misdiagnosing transient (and/or rate-related) AV dissociation as complete AV block.

<u>Practice</u>: *Why is this not 3° AV block?*

Use the **4 *Question Approach*** to interpret the rhythm shown below.

> <u>HINT</u>- Resist the urge to comment on the dropped beats that are seen in
> the initial part of the tracing- until you have *systematically* analyzed
> the rest of the tracing!

Lead MCL$_1$

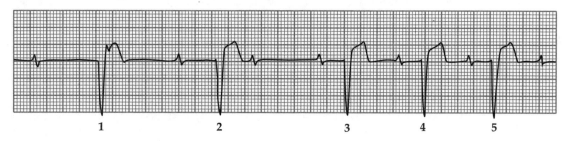

<u>Additional Question</u> → Which of the criteria required for diagnosis of 3° AV block are *not* present in this tracing? (Feel free to refer
to page 250 in formulating your answer.)

Interpretation:

Applying the **4 Question Approach** to the rhythm that appears on page 251- we note the following:

i) The *width* of the QRS complex is at the upper limit of normal. That is, the QRS is about *half* a large box (or 0.10 second) in duration.

ii) The ventricular rhythm is clearly *not* regular. As emphasized on page 250- *recognition of this fact should immediately suggest that the rhythm is not 3° AV block.*

iii) P waves are definitely present. The *atrial* rhythm (P-P interval) is almost regular (although there is *some* variation that is most likely due to *ventriculophasic sinus arrhythmia*- as described on page 246).

iv) Some P waves are related to neighboring QRS complexes. *Others are not.*

Comment → The *KEY* to interpreting this complicated rhythm lies with assessing the last component of the **4 Question Approach**- which relates to determining if a relationship exists between P waves and neighboring QRS complexes. Early on in this tracing there is no such relationship. P waves occurring during this initial part of the tracing are completely *unrelated* to the QRS complex. Early on then (i.e., for beats #1 and #2) there is *AV dissociation.* However, this changes for the last three beats on the tracing. That is, beats #3, 4, and 5 all appear to be sinus conducted- as evidenced by a PR interval that is *fixed* (albeit *prolonged* to 0.30 second). Thus, the underlying rhythm that appears on page 251 is **sinus** with **1° AV block**. There is *transient* **AV dissociation** early on in the tracing (although the reason for this AV dissociation is unclear). The point to emphasize is that 3° AV block is *not* present- since the ventricular response is *not* regular, and the last three beats on the tracing *are* conducted. (Instead we suspect that a more complex form of 2° AV block is probably present).

AV Dissociation

- *Definition/Clinical Application* -

Perhaps the area that causes the greatest confusion regarding the AV blocks concerns the term *AV dissociation*. Expanding upon the brief description we cited on page 244, we favor the following clinical defintion:

> *AV dissociation* is a *secondary* rhythm disturbance (*never* a primary disturbance) that occurs when the atria and ventricles *fail* to respond to same impulse. The result is that atria and ventricles beat *independently* of each other.

KEY → One should *never* say that a rhythm "is" AV dissociation- but rather that AV dissociation is present because of _____ (= the *primary* disorder).

Clinically there are *three* reasons why AV dissociation may develop. *Can you think of what they might be?*

The 3 Causes of AV Dissociation:

1. *"Default"*- from *slowing* of the sinus pacemaker.

2. *"Usurpation"*- from *acceleration* of a junctional or ventricular focus that speeeds up and *takes over* (i.e., "usurps") the primary pacemaking function.

3. *AV block*- which produces slowing of the ventricular response by preventing conduction of one or more sinus impulses.

KEY → Several points should be emphasized regarding the phenomenon of **AV dissociation**. They include:

- that AV block is only one of the conditions that can cause AV dissociation. The other two conditions that can cause AV dissociation are *usurpation* and *default*.

- that AV dissociation is *not* the same as 3° (complete) AV block. *It can't be*- since other conditions (i.e., usurpation, default and/or 2° AV block) may also cause AV dissociation.

- that AV dissociation may either be *short-lived* (occurring for only a few beats as in the rhythm shown on page 251)- or much longer lasting. With 3° AV block, AV dissociation is persistent (i.e., "complete")- so that *none* of the atrial impulses are conducted to the ventricles.

- that recognition of AV dissociation (even if prolonged) does *not* necessarily mean that any heart block at all is present! AV dissociation per se need *not* necessarily be treated- especially if the cause is benign and the patient is hemodynamically stable.

AV Dissociation

- *AV Dissociation by Default* -

Use the **4 Question Approach** to interpret the rhythm shown below.

> <u>HINT</u>- Be sure to consider the *KEY* on the front of page 253 in formulating your answer.

Lead II

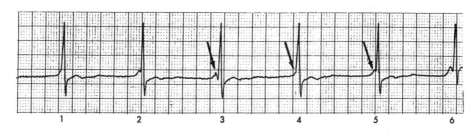

Additional Questions:

1. Why would it be wrong to interpret the above rhythm as 3° AV block?

> <u>HINT</u>- Do P waves in this tracing (*arrows*) have a *chance* to conduct?

2. Can you say that any degree of AV block at all is present in the above tracing?

Interpretation:

Applying the **4 *Question Approach*** to the rhythm that appears on page 255- we note the following:

i) The QRS complex is *narrow* (i.e., not more than *half* a large box in duration).

ii) The ventricular rhythm is almost precisely *regular*- with an R-R interval that is slighty less than 6 large boxes in duration (which corresponds to a heart rate of **53 beats/minute**).

iii) & iv) Atrial activity *is* present! P waves precede each QRS complex and deform the initial upstroke (*arrows* in the Figure). However- *none* of the P waves are related in any consistent manner to the QRS complex (i.e., the PR interval is extremely short and keeps changing). This means that **complete AV dissociation** must therefore be present.

> **Comment** → As emphasized in the *KEY* on page 253- AV dissociation is *never* a diagnosis. Instead, it is *always* secondary to something else. In this case the *underlying* rhythm is sinus bradycardia. Because of progressive slowing of the atrial rate (i.e., *"default"* of the sinus pacemaker)- the natural response of the AV node (as the "next pacemaker in line")- is to emit an *escape* rhythm in the hope of preventing excessive bradycardia. Thus, our interpretation of this rhythm would be **sinus bradycardia** (our *primary* diagnosis)- which produces **AV dissociation** (in this case by *default*)- with emergence of an appropriate **AV nodal *escape* rhythm**.

> **KEY** → The point to emphasize is that *despite* the presence of *complete* AV dissociation- the rhythm on the front of this card does *not* represent complete AV block! This is because *none* of the P waves are ever given a *chance* to conduct (because the PR interval is always too short!). Although some form of AV block *may* be present- there is simply *no way to tell* from the short rhythm strip shown if P waves *could* conduct- *were they given the chance.*

AV Dissociation

- *AV Dissociation by Usurpation* -

Use the **4 Question Approach** to interpret the rhythm shown below.

Lead MCL₁

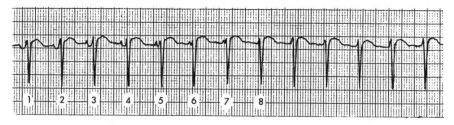

Additional Questions:

1. Are P waves conducting for the *first few beats* in the above tracing? Do you *also* think the P waves preceding beats #5, 6, and 7 are conducting?

2. Does the rhythm shown above represent 3° AV block? *Can you say that there is any AV block at all?*

    <u>HINT</u>- Do the P waves that fail to conduct have a *chance* to conduct?

Interpretation:

Applying the **4 *Question Approach*** to the rhythm that appears on page 257- we note the following:

i) & ii) The QRS complex is *narrow* (i.e., not more than *half* a large box in duration). The ventricular (QRS) rhythm is *regular* at a rate of approximately 115 beats/minute.

iii) & iv) Atrial activity *is* present- at least for a portion of this tracing. P waves clearly precede the first few beats- but become lost after beat #7. Although admittedly the PR interval is relatively short for beats #1-4 (i.e., about 0.10 second)- the constant PR interval suggests that these first few beats are probably still conducting. However, the P waves preceding beats #5, 6, and 7 are definitely *not* conducting- because the PR interval becomes far too short. Thus, **AV dissociation** must be present- at least *temporarily* (since P waves are at least temporarily *unrelated* to QRS complexes). This means that a *junctional* rhythm must be present (at least on latter part of the tracing)- since the ventricular rhythm is regular, P waves are absent, and the QRS complex is narrow and identical to the QRS of the first few sinus beats.

> **Comment** → This is a complex rhythm strip. Nevertheless, the correct interpretation can be systematically arrived at by synthesizing the findings described above. **Sinus tachycardia** is probably present for the first few beats in the tracing. Thereafter there is **AV dissociation**- in this case as a result of *usurpation* (as described on page 254) from an *accelerated* junctional pacemaker that takes over the pacemaking function. As noted on pages 147-148- the conditions most commonly associated with **junctional tachycardia** are digitalis toxicity, acute inferior infarction, and the post-operative state.
>
> The point to emphasize is that we simply can *not* tell from this short rhythm strip if any AV block is present at all. This is because despite the presence of AV dissociation- P waves are *never* shown to fail to conduct at a time when they should conduct.

<u>High Grade AV Block</u>

- *Why is this <u>not</u> 3° (complete) AV block?* -

Use the **4 *Question Approach*** to interpret the rhythm shown below. Note that we have *already* seen this tracing (on page 85).

Lead II

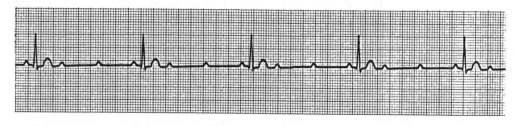

<u>Additional Questions:</u>

1. Despite the fact that most P waves in the above tracing are "dropped" (i.e., *not* conducting)- this rhythm is *not* 3° AV block. *Why not?*

   <u>HINT</u>- Do at least *some* P waves conduct?

2. What *degree* of AV block *is* present?

Answer:

Applying the **4 Question Approach** to the rhythm that appears on page 259- we note the following:

i) P waves *are* present throughout the tracing.

ii) The QRS complex is *narrow* (i.e., clearly *not* more than *half* a large box in duration).

iii) The rhythm is *regular*. This holds true for *both* the P wave rhythm (since the P-P interval is constant)- as well as for the ventricular rhythm (since the R-R interval is also constant). The P-P interval is slightly *less* than 3 large boxes in duration- which corresponds to an *atrial* rate of about 105 beats/minute. The R-R interval is between 8 to 9 large boxes in duration- which corresponds to a *ventricular* rate of about 35 beats/minute.

iv) There *is* a relation between P waves and the QRS complex. That is- *each* QRS complex in the tracing *is* preceded by a P wave- and the PR interval that precedes each QRS is *fixed* (i.e., constant). However, many P waves are *not* followed by a QRS- so that *only* one out of every three P waves is conducted to the ventricles (i.e., there is **3:1 AV conduction**).

Comment → Application of the *'KISS Method'* (described on page 240)- suggests that the rhythm on page 259 must represent a form of **2° AV block**. We say this because it is clear that *some* degree of AV block must be present (since some P waves that should be conducting are *not* conducting)- yet the rhythm is definitely *not* 1° AV block- nor 3° AV block. No P waves at all should conduct if 3° AV block was present. By the process of elimination, the rhythm must therefore represent some form of 2° AV block. Because *several* P waves are dropped for each one that is conducted- we describe this rhythm as representing **high grade** *(or high degree)* **AV block**.

2° AV Block

- Definition/Types of 2° AV Block -

As suggested on page 236- 2° AV block is said to be present when some atrial impulses are being conducted to the ventricles- *but others are not (as a result of AV block).*

Traditionally, two types of 2° AV block are usually described: Mobitz type I and Mobitz type II. We favor slight modification of this *traditional* classification- with addition of a *third* category of 2° AV block:

Modified Classification of the AV Blocks:

- *1° AV Block*

- *2° AV Block* :
    - Mobitz type I (= Wenckebach)
    - Mobitz type II
    - 2° AV block with 2:1 AV conduction

- *3° (= Complete) AV Block*

KEY → Unless underlying sinus arrhythmia is present- the *atrial* rate should be *regular* (or at least *almost* regular) with 2° AV block! Awareness of this point is invaluable in helping to distinguish between *true* 2° AV block (in one of its various forms)- from *mimics* of 2° AV block (such as blocked PACs and sinus pauses).

Modified Classification of 2° AV Block

- **Mobitz I (Wenckebach)** - the most common form of 2° AV block (*by far!*)- in which the PR interval *progressively lengthens* until a beat is dropped (*See pages 263-268*).

- **Mobitz II** - the much less common (and more severe) form of 2° AV block- in which there is *failed* conduction of atrial impulses following *consecutively* conducted beats that manifest a *constant* PR interval (*See pages 275-276*).

- **2° AV block with 2:1 AV conduction** - the diagnostically problematic form of 2° AV block- because definitive differentiation between Mobitz type I and Mobitz type II may *not* be possible (*See pages 279-280*).

Note → It is important to always consider the *appropriateness* of the failed conduction. For example, it's actually a *blessing* (and *not* a manifestation of AV block) that the AV node does not allow 1:1 AV conduction in the presence of **atrial flutter** when the atrial rate approaches 300 beats/minute. If every atrial impulse was to be conducted in this situation- then the ventricular response would be 300 beats/minute- a rate that is far *too fast* to allow adequate ventricular filling. It is precisely for this reason that we describe the rhythm shown in the top panel of page 115 as **atrial flutter** with **2:1 AV conduction**- rather than with the term 2:1 AV "block".

2° AV Block

- *Mobitz Type I (Wenckebach)* -

Use the **4 Question Approach** to interpret the rhythm shown below.

<u>HINT</u>- What happens to the PR interval with successive beats?

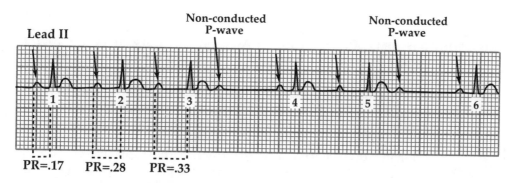

Additional Questions:

1. Is the atrial rhythm regular?

2. Is the ventricular rhythm regular?

Interpretation:

Applying the *4 Question Approach* to the rhythm that appears on page 263- we note the following:

    i) P waves *are* present throughout the tracing (*arrows*). The atrial rhythm is regular- with a P-P interval of 3 large boxes in duration (which corresponds to an *atrial* rate of 100/minute).

    ii) & iii) The QRS complex is *narrow* (i.e., clearly *not* more than *half* a large box in duration). Unlike the atrial rhythm- the ventricular rhythm is *not* regular.

    iv) The PR interval continually changes. Despite this- there *is* a relationship between P waves and the QRS complex (*See Comment below*).

Comment → As is often the case for AV conduction disorders- the *KEY* to interpreting the rhythm lies with assessing the *last* component of the *4 Question Approach*. This relates to determining whether a relationship exists between P waves and neighboring QRS complexes. The best way to do this is to focus attention on *each* QRS complex in the tracing- and then to determine the PR interval between that QRS and the P wave that *precedes* it.

    Applying this approach to the rhythm that appears on page 263- it can be seen that the PR interval *progressively* increases for the first 3 beats in this tracing (i.e., from 0.17- to 0.28- to 0.33 second)- until finally the P wave that follows beat #3 is "dropped" (i.e., *not* conducted). The cycle then resumes with shortening of the PR interval preceding beat #4- lengthening of the next PR interval- and then *non-conduction* of the P wave that follows beat #5. This *relationship*- of a progressively lengthening PR interval until a beat is dropped- defines the rhythm on the front of this card as **2° AV block** of the **Mobitz I (Wenckebach) type**.

Group Beating

- *The "Footprints" of Wenckebach* -

Use the **4 Question Approach** to interpret the rhythm shown below.

> <u>HINT</u>- Is there a *pattern* to the regularity of the ventricular response in the rhythm below? (Feel free to refer back to pages 65-66 in formulating your answer.)

Lead II

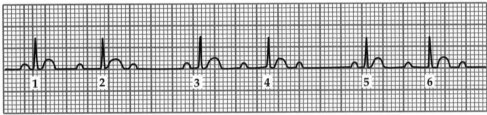

<u>**Additional Questions**</u> → What are the characteristic features (i.e., *"footprints"*) of Wenckebach-type conduction disorders? *How many of these features can you identify in the above tracing?*

Interpretation:

Applying the **4 *Question Approach*** to the rhythm that appears on page 265- we note the following:

i) P waves *are* present throughout the tracing. The atrial rhythm is fairly regular- with a P-P interval of between 2 and 3 large boxes in duration (which corresponds to an *atrial* rate of ≈115/minute).

ii) The QRS complex is *narrow* (i.e., clearly *not* more than *half* a large box in duration).

iii) The ventricular rhythm is *not* regular. Despite this- there *is* a pattern to the ventricular beats. As suggested in the note on page 66- it is sometimes easiest to recognize the overall pattern of rhythm regularity by **stepping back** a short distance from the tracing being examined. *Try this yourself-* especially if you have not yet appreciated the pattern of **"group beating"** for the rhythm that appears on page 265. Three "groups" (of two beats each) should be recognized (i.e., beats #1-2; 3-4; and 5-6).

iv) The PR interval is definitely *not* constant. As was the case for the rhythm on page 263- *despite* this changing PR interval, there *is* a relationship between P waves and the QRS complex (*See Comment below*).

Comment → The rhythm that appears on page 265 represents **2° AV block, Mobitz type I** (= Wenckebach)- in this case with **3:2 AV conduction** (since there are three P waves for every two QRS complexes that are conducted). The three most characteristic features (i.e., **"footprints"**) of 2° AV Wenckebach are all present in this tracing: **1)** group beating; **2)** regularity of the atrial rate; and **3)** progressive lengthening of the PR interval until a beat is dropped. In addition, the QRS complex is *narrow* (as it most often is with this form of 2° AV block).

Wenckebach Blocks

- A closer look at the "Footprints" -

As suggested by our discussion of the rhythm shown on page 265- 2° AV block, Mobitz type I is characterized by a number of findings that are affectionately known as the ***"Footprints of Wenckebach"*** (Marriott). In addition to the three *"footprints"* that were noted on page 266- we add two new features:

The "Footprints" of Wenckebach:

1. *Group beating.*
2. *Regularity* of the atrial rate.
3. Progressive *lengthening* of the PR interval until a beat is dropped.
4. Duration of the pause (that contains the dropped beat) of *less* than twice the shortest R-R interval.
5. Progressive *shortening* of the R-R interval *within* groups of beats.

Note → Not all of the *footprints* need to be present in every example of Wenckebach. By way of illustration- return to the rhythm that was shown on page 263. Four of the *footprints* are seen in this example. That is, the *atrial* rate is regular- the PR interval progressively *increases* until a beat is dropped (from 0.17- to 0.28- to 0.33 second)- the pause containing the dropped beat (i.e., the interval between beats #3-4) is *less* than twice the shortest R-R interval (which is the R-R interval between beats #2-3)- and the R-R interval *shortens* within the first group of beats (i.e., the R-R interval between beats #2-3 is *shorter* than the R-R interval between beats #1-2).

The one *footprint* that is *not* well appreciated in this example is group beating- although it is possible that this might be seen if a longer rhythm strip was available.

Clinical Utility of the "Footprints" of Wenckebach

The term **"Wenckebach"** is falsely assumed by many health care providers to be synonymous with 2° AV block, Mobitz type I. Actually, there are *many* different types of *"Wenckebach-like"* conduction disturbances- of which 2° AV Wenckebach is only one form. Other less commonly occurring examples include SA Wenckebach, Wenckebach AV conduction in the presence of atrial fibrillation or atrial flutter, VT or junctional rhythm with *retrograde* Wenckebach- and many more! Although in-depth discussion of these Wenckebach phenomena clearly extends *beyond* the scope of this book- the clinical point to emphasize is that recognition of the typical "footprints" of **Wenckebach periodicity** should prompt suspicion of the presence of this conduction disturbance- *even when P waves are absent* !

PEARL → *KEY* features about specific footprints are noted below:

- **Group Beating-** is the hallmark of Wenckebach conduction (and often provides the very *first* clue that this conduction disturbance may be present. As suggested on page 266- group beating is usually best seen by *stepping back* a short distance from the tracing. Yet as helpful to diagnosis as recognizing group beating is- we caution that all group beating is *not* necessarily the result of Wenckebach conduction (*See page 273*).

- **Regularity of the Atrial Rate-** is important for ruling out *other* causes of group beating (such as marked sinus arrhythmia, atrial bigeminy or trigeminy, blocked PACs, sinus exit blocks, etc.).

- **Wenckebach Periodicity-** is suggested by progressive *lengthening* of the PR interval- progressive *shortening* of the R-R interval *within* groups of beats- and duration of the pause (containing the dropped beat) that is *less* than twice the shortest R-R interval.

<u>Practice</u>: *Is this Wenckebach?*

The tracing below was obtained from a patient in atrial fibrillation who was being treated with digoxin. Despite the fact that P waves are absent (because the rhythm is atrial fibrillation)- there *is* evidence of *Wenckebach-type* conduction. *Why do we say this?*

> <u>HINT #1</u>- Feel free to refer to pages 267-268 in formulating your answer.
>
> <u>HINT #2</u>- You may want to *step back* a short distance to view the tracing.
>
> <u>HINT #3</u>- Remember that *not* all of the footprints need always be present for there to be Wenckebach conduction.

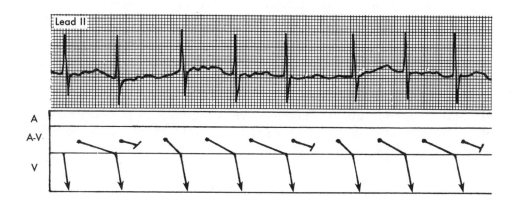

Answer:

The rhythm that appears on page 269 is *not* a simple tracing. Nevertheless, we hope that you recognized the presence of ***group beating***.

The pattern can probably best be appreciated by viewing the tracing from a short distance away. After the initial two beats in the tracing comes a short pause- followed by the *first* group of 3 beats- followed by another short pause- and then the *second* group of 3 beats. *If all you did was to recognize the presence of this regular irregularity (i.e., group beating)-* then you will have accomplished our objective for this tracing. If you went one step further and said that the presence of group beating makes it likely that *some* type of Wenckebach conduction is operative- you will have captured the essence of the concept we are stressing.

Beyond the Core → Further interpretation of this tracing reveals that the QRS complex is *narrow*- which suggests a *supraventricular* mechanism for the rhythm. P waves are absent in this lead II monitoring lead. Instead, fine undulations are seen in the baseline. These findings are consistent with the fact that the *underlying* rhythm is still atrial fibrillation.

The *laddergram* seen below the rhythm provides an explanation for the group beating. This patient had digitalis toxicity- which produced complete (3°) AV block. As a result, *none* of the fibrillatory atrial impulses were able to penetrate the AV node. The patient responded with an accelerated junctional escape rhythm and Wenckebach conduction *out of* the AV node- which produced characteristic *Wenckebach periodicity* of the ventricular response (with group beating, shortening of the R-R interval within groups of beats, and pause duration of *less* than twice the shortest R-R interval).

KEY → Full understanding of the mechanism of this rhythm is an advanced concept that clearly extends beyond the scope of this book. Our principal objective is simply to have you recognize the group beating *pattern* to the ventricular response- and to realize that *despite* the presence of atrial fibrillation, a Wenckebach block is still likely to be present.

Practice: *Is this Wenckebach?*

Use the **4 Question Approach** to interpret the rhythm shown below.

> <u>HINT</u>- *What happens to the PR interval?* Be sure to specifically look at the PR interval of the beat *just before* the pause (i.e., of beat #8)- and to *compare* this to the PR interval at the beginning of the rhythm strip- *as well as* to the PR interval at the *end* of the pause (i.e., the PR interval of beat #9).

Lead II

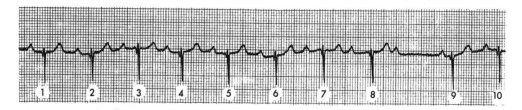

<u>**Additional Question**</u> → Do you recognize any *"footprints"* of *Wenckebach* in the above tracing? If so- *which ones?* (Feel free to refer to page 267 in formulating your answer.)

Interpretation:

Applying the **4 *Question Approach*** to the rhythm that appears on page 271- we note the following:

i) P waves *are* present throughout the tracing. The atrial rhythm is fairly regular- with a P-P interval of between 3 and 4 large boxes in duration (which corresponds to an *atrial* rate of about 85/minute).

ii) & iii) The QRS complex appears to be *narrow* (i.e., *not* more than *half* a large box in duration). The ventricular rhythm is *not* regular (since a definite *pause* interrupts the rhythm after beat #8).

iv) It is difficult to tell from initial inspection if a relationship exists between P waves and neighboring QRS complexes (*See Comment below*).

> **Comment** → It appears that the first 8 beats in this tracing on page 271 are **sinus** conducted with **1° AV block**. If one merely compared consecutive PR intervals during these 8 conducted beats- it would *not* be immediately apparent that the PR interval was progressively lengthening. Only by comparing the PR interval of the beat *just before* the pause (i.e., the PR interval of beat #8)- with the PR interval at the start of the rhythm strip (i.e., the PR interval of beat #1)- can it be readily seen that the PR interval must be increasing. Note that the PR interval shortens again with beat #9- which signals the onset of the next Wenckebach cycle.

KEY → The diagnosis of **2° AV block, Mobitz type I** (Wenckebach) is made for this rhythm on the basis of *regularity* of the atrial rate in association with the finding of **Wenckebach periodicity** (including lengthening PR interval- and pause duration of *less* than twice the shortest R-R interval).

All Group Beating ≠ Wenckebach

Despite the presence of group beating in each of the three rhythms shown below- *none* of these rhythms represent 2° AV Wenckebach. *Can you identify the cause of group beating in each case?*

> <u>HINT</u>- Pay particular attention to the morphology and *regularity* of the atrial response (and/or the *lack* thereof).

Lead II

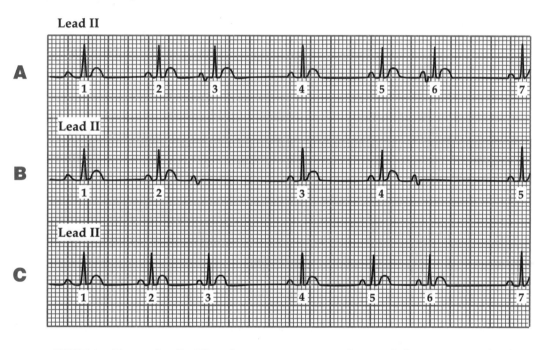

> <u>HINT to Example C</u>- This last tracing was obtained from a completely healthy young child.

All Group Beating ≠ Wenckebach

Although the presence of **group beating** should always suggest the *possibility* of Wenckebach conduction- *other* conditions may also produce this phenomenon. Distinction between *true* Wenckebach- and *other* conditions that produce group beating can be greatly facilitated using the *"footprints"* (that were described on page 267). Regarding the tracings that appear on page 273:

- *Example A*- is *not* Wenckebach because the PR interval is not increasing and the atrial rate is not regular. Instead, every third P wave looks different (i.e., is biphasic) and occurs early. Thus, the *underlying* rhythm is **sinus**- and beats #3 and #6 are **PACs**. The reason for *group beating* in this tracing is **atrial trigeminy** (i.e., every *third* beat is a PAC).

- *Example B*- is *not* Wenckebach because once again the PR interval is not increasing (for consecutively conducted beats)- and the atrial rate is not regular. Instead, every third P wave occurs early- looks different- and is *not* followed by a QRS complex (i.e., the PACs that follow beats #2 and #4 are *blocked*). Once again, the rhythm is **sinus** with **atrial trigeminy**- however this time, every third beat is a *non-conducted* PAC.

> Clinically, it is extremely helpful to remember- **the *most common* cause of a pause** (*by far!*) is a **blocked PAC** (and *not* AV block!).

- *Example C*- is *not* Wenckebach because the PR interval is not increasing, and the atrial rate is not regular. Instead- each QRS is preceded by a normal appearing P wave with a *constant* PR interval. The rhythm is **sinus arrhythmia**- which is an extremely common normal finding among children and young adults (in whom heart rate *often* varies in cyclical fashion according to the pattern of respiration).

> ***Beyond the Core (!)*** Another possible explanation for the group beating seen in Example C is SA nodal exit block (SA Wenckebach)- although this uncommon (and difficult to diagnose) form of SA block should *not* be expected in a healthy child.

2° AV Block

- *Mobitz Type II* -

Use the **4 Question Approach** to interpret the rhythm shown below.

<u>HINT</u>- What happens to the PR interval with *consecutively conducted* beats?

Lead II

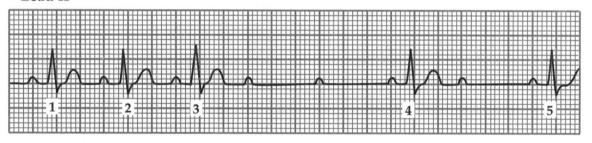

<u>Additional Questions:</u>

1. Is the atrial rate regular?

2. Is the ventricular rate regular?

Interpretation:

Applying the **4 *Question Approach*** to the rhythm that appears on page 275- we note the following:

   i) P waves *are* present throughout the tracing. The atrial rhythm is regular- with a P-P interval of 3 large boxes in duration (which corresponds to an *atrial* rate of 100/minute).

   ii) & iii) The QRS complex is *wide* (i.e., clearly *more* than *half* a large box in duration). Unlike the atrial rhythm- the ventricular rhythm is *not* regular.

   iv) A relationship *does* exist between P waves and neighboring QRS complexes. The best way to establish this relationship is to focus attention on *each* QRS complex in the tracing. Then look to identify the P wave that immediately precedes it- and determine if the PR interval is constant. It should be apparent that beats #1, 2, 3- as well as #4 and 5 are *all* preceded by P waves that manifest a *fixed* PR interval- which suggests that these P waves *are* conducting.

Comment → The rhythm that appears on page 275 clearly represents some form of AV block. We say this with certainty because *unlike* the rhythms that were shown on page 273- P wave morphology in this tracing remains constant throughout and the atrial rate remains regular. These findings essentially *rule out* the mimics of AV block such as PACs, sinus arrhythmia, sinus pauses and sinus exit block.

   The conduction disturbance is clearly *not* simple 1° AV block. It is also definitely *not* complete (3°) AV block- because we know that at least *some* P waves *are* conducting (as evidenced by the constant PR interval before beats #1, 2, and 3). This means that the rhythm must represent a form of 2° AV block. As defined on page 262- the presence of QRS widening and a *constant* PR interval for *consecutively conducted* beats until one or more beats are dropped identifies this rhythm as **2° AV block, Mobitz type II.**

<u>2° AV Block:</u> Mobitz I vs. Mobitz II

- *Anatomic Level/Clinical Implications* -

The major clinical implications of Mobitz I and Mobitz II 2° AV block are easily remembered if one keeps in mind the usual *anatomic* site of each of these conduction disorders:

- **Mobitz I** - usually occurs **_at_** the level of the AV node
- **Mobitz II** - usually occurs **_below_** the level of the AV node.

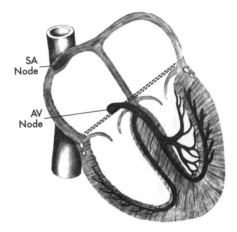

<u>KEY Clinical Questions:</u>

1. What would you expect the QRS complex to look like for **Mobitz II** 2° AV block- given that the anatomic level of this block almost always originates *below* the double dotted line in the above Figure?

2. Which conduction defect would you expect to be more severe- Mobitz I or Mobitz II? Which one occurs more commonly in clinical practice?

2° AV Block- *Mobitz I or Mobitz II?*

- **_Mobitz I_**- is most often associated with acute *inferior* infarction. Anatomically, the site of this block is usually located **_at_** the level of the AV node. This accounts for the fact that the QRS complex will usually be *narrow*. The PR interval may be prolonged (producing 1° AV block)- because of impaired conduction through the AV node. Clinically- because the level of block is *higher* in the conduction system, the resultant rhythm is generally much more reliable than it is with Mobitz II. The patient is therefore more likely to be asymptomatic and hemodynamically stable- so that close observation (until the conduction disturbance spontaneously resolves) may be all that is needed. If hemodynamic status becomes compromised (due to marked bradycardia)- atropine will often be effective in improving AV conduction (since the level of block is *at* the AV node). Pacemaker therapy is rarely needed.

- **_Mobitz II_**- is usually associated with acute *anterior* (or anteroseptal) myocardial infarction. The level of this block is anatomically *lower* in the conduction system than it is for Mobitz I (i.e., the level of block is **_below_** the AV node). As a result, the QRS complex is most often *wide*- and the resulting rhythm much *less* reliable. Mobitz II has a most disturbing tendency to rapidly progress from trivial block (dropping only occasional beats) to *complete* AV block- or even *ventricular standstill* (which sometimes occurs with little or no warning). *Immediate* consideration of pacemaker therapy is therefore essential as soon as this conduction disturbance is recognized. This is in contrast to Mobitz I which tends to occur as part of an *orderly* progression (i.e., from 1° to 2° to 3° AV block) in those cases of acute inferior infarction in which complete AV block does develop. Because of the low (*infranodal*) anatomic level of the conduction disturbance with Mobitz II- atropine will rarely be effective in improving the ventricular response.

Note → Mobitz I 2° AV block is much, much more common in clinical practice than Mobitz II. (It is likely that more than 90% of 2° AV block is the result of Mobitz I).

2:1 AV Conduction

- *Mobitz I or Mobitz II ???* -

Use the **4 *Question Approach*** to interpret the rhythm shown below.

Lead II

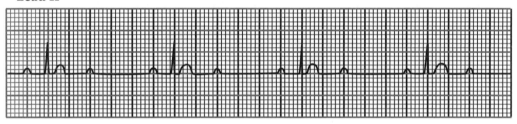

Additional Questions:

1. Is the rhythm shown above more likely to represent 2° AV block, Mobitz type II (because the PR interval is fixed)- or Mobitz I? *Are you able to tell for sure?*

 HINT- Does this tracing provide you with *enough information* to tell if the PR interval is lengthening?

2. What factors are in favor of the rhythm being Mobitz I? (Feel free to refer to page 278 in formulating your answer.)

Interpretation:

Applying the *4 Question Approach* to the rhythm that appears on page 279- we note the following:

i) P waves *are* present throughout the tracing. The atrial rhythm is regular- with a P-P interval of 3 large boxes in duration (which corresponds to an *atrial* rate of 100/minute).

ii) & iii) The QRS complex is *narrow* (i.e., *not* more than *half* a large box in duration). The ventricular rhythm is regular- with an R-R interval of 6 large boxes in duration (which corresponds to a rate of 50 beats/minute).

iv) A relationship *does* exist between P waves and neighboring QRS complexes. Focusing attention on *each* QRS complex in the tracing- it can be seen that a P wave immediately *precedes* each QRS- and that the PR interval of this preceding P wave is constant. This suggests that these P waves *are* conducting. However- *every other P wave* is blocked (i.e., *non-conducted*)- so that there is **2:1 AV block**.

Comment → The rhythm shown on page 279 represents **2° AV block**- in this case with **2:1 AV conduction**. As described on page 262- this is the diagnostically problematic form of 2° AV block. Because consecutively conducted beats do *not* occur- it is *impossible* to determine if the PR interval is "lengthening" (i.e., since you *never* see two beats occur in a row). One therefore *can't* be certain about whether this rhythm represents Mobitz I or Mobitz II. Factors in favor of **Mobitz I** are the *narrow* QRS complex- and the statistical fact that Mobitz I is far more common than Mobitz II (See page 278). A more subtle additional point in favor of Mobitz I is that those P waves that do conduct- do so with 1° AV block.

Practice: *Mobitz I or Mobitz II ?*

As emphasized in the Comment on page 280- it is often difficult to distinguish between Mobitz I and Mobitz II 2° AV block when there is 2:1 AV conduction. In addition to the differentiating features described on page 278- it may be helpful to remember that it is highly *unlikely* for a patient to switch back and forth from Mobitz I to Mobitz II. Therefore- if *elsewhere* on the tracing (and/or on prior tracings) there is clear evidence of Mobitz I- the chances are excellent that the 2:1 AV conduction is *also* a manifestation of Mobitz I. *Apply this information to the rhythm shown below.* Which type of 2° AV block is more likely- Mobitz I or Mobitz II?

> <u>HINT</u>- Resist the urge to commit to an answer until you have analyzed the last two beats in the tracing! (Be sure to note what happens to the PR interval when *consecutively* conducted beats *are* seen.)

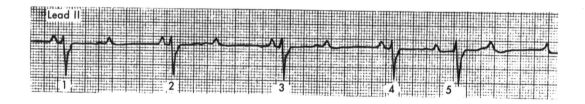

Additional Question → How would you have interpreted this
rhythm strip if the tracing had ended *after* beat #4 ???

Answer:

Although admittedly it is difficult to be certain of where the QRS complex ends and the ST segment begins- the QRS in this tracing appears to be slightly prolonged (i.e., it appears to be *more* than *half* a large box in duration). The ventricular rhythm is *not* completely regular. However, the atrial rhythm is regular- with a P-P interval of about 4 large boxes in duration (which corresponds to an *atrial* rate of about 75/minute).

Close inspection of the first four beats in the tracing reveals that every other P wave is blocked. For those P waves that *are* conducted (to produce beats #1, 2, 3, and 4)- the PR interval preceding each QRS remains constant. If the rhythm strip were to end here (i.e., *after* beat #4)- the tracing would have to be interpreted as representing 2° AV block with 2:1 AV conduction. In this situation, it would be *impossible* to distinguish between Mobitz I and Mobitz II- although because of QRS widening, one would have to be concerned about the possibility of Mobitz II.

As emphasized on page 262- *definitive* differentiation between Mobitz I and Mobitz II may not be possible in the setting of 2° AV block when there is *pure* 2:1 AV conduction. This is *not* the case here, however- since the *telltale* sign of *Wenckebach* (which is PR interval lengthening) surfaces at the end of the tracing. That is- the PR interval preceding beat #5 *lengthens* with respect to the PR interval preceding beat #4. Because it is exceedingly unlikely for a patient to switch abruptly from Mobitz I to Mobitz II- the conduction disturbance that is shown on page 281 almost certainly represents **2° AV block** of the **Mobitz I type** (here with 2:1 and 3:2 AV conduction)- and *not* Mobitz II!

> **KEY** → As suggested on page 262- one should think of the **2° AV blocks** as occurring in one of *three* clinical forms: 1) *definitely* Mobitz I; 2) *definitely* Mobitz II; or 3) **2:1 AV conduction-** *in which case you can't always be sure* !

<u>Review</u>: *Is there AV block ?*

Use the **4 *Question Approach*** to interpret the rhythm shown below. *Is there AV block?* If so- *which type?*

Lead MCL$_1$

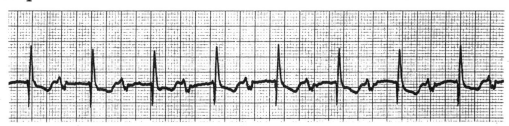

<u>Additional Question</u> → The QRS complex appears to be slightly
widened. *Why might this be ?*

Interpretation:

Applying the **4 *Question Approach*** to the rhythm that appears on page 283- we note the following:

    i) & ii) As suggested in the *Additional Question-* the QRS complex appears to be slightly *widened.* The ventricular rhythm is *regular-* with an R-R interval of just over 4 large boxes in duration (which corresponds to a rate of about 70 beats/minute).

    iii) & iv) P waves *are* present. Focusing attention on *each* QRS complex- it can be seen that a P wave immediately *precedes* each QRS- and is *related* to that QRS by a *fixed* (albeit markedly prolonged) PR interval (of 0.41 second).

Comment → The rhythm that appears on page 283 is **sinus-** since each QRS complex in the tracing is preceded by a P wave with a fixed PR interval. In addition, there is **1° AV block**. The reason for QRS widening is *preexisting* right bundle branch block (rSR' pattern in this right-sided monitoring lead).

<u>Review</u>: *Is there AV block ?*

Use the **4 *Question Approach*** to interpret the rhythm shown below. *Is there AV block?* If so- *which type?*

> <u>HINT</u>- What helpful clue to the etiology of this rhythm might you see best from a distance *away* (i.e., "from the *back* of the room") ???

Lead MCL₁

Lead MCL_1

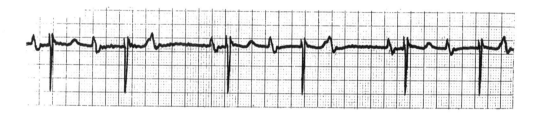

<u>Additional Question</u> → How many *"footprints"* are present in the above tracing?

Interpretation:

Regarding the rhythm that appears on page 285- the helpful clue that can best be seen "from the *back* of the room" is the presence of ***group beating*** (in this case with *three* groups of *two* beats each). Recognition of this finding should always suggest the *possibility* of a Wenckebach-type conduction disorder. Awareness of this possibility may be extremely helpful as one systematically proceeds with interpretation. Using the **4 *Question Approach***- we note the following:

i) P waves *are* present throughout the tracing. Use of calipers facilitates recognition of the *third*- *sixth*- and *ninth* P waves- each of which is partially hidden within the T wave of the preceding QRS complex. Note that the atrial rhythm is fairly regular- with a P-P interval of between 4 and 5 large boxes in duration (which corresponds to an *atrial* rate of about 65-70 beats/minute).

ii) & iii) The QRS complex is *narrow* (i.e., *not* more than *half* a large box in duration). However- the ventricular rhythm is *not* regular.

iv) P waves *are* related to neighboring QRS complexes. Focusing attention on *each* QRS in the tracing- it can be seen that a P wave *precedes* each QRS- and is *related* to that QRS by progressive *lengthening* of the PR interval (from 0.24 to 0.48 second) *within* each group of beats- until a beat is dropped.

> **Comment** → The rhythm that appears on page 285 represents a form of **2° AV block**. Recognition of *group beating* suggests at the outset that this may be AV Wenckebach (Mobitz I). Systematic interpretation as described above reveals the presence of most of the other **"*footprints*"** listed on pages 267-268- including *regularity* of the atrial rate- progressive *lengthening* of the PR interval until a beat is dropped- and duration of the pause (that contains the dropped beat) of *less* than twice the shortest R-R interval. This confirms our impression that this rhythm is 2° AV block, **Mobitz type I**- in this case with 3:2 AV conduction.

<u>Review</u>: *Is there AV block ?*

Use the **4 Question Approach** to interpret the rhythm shown below. *Is there AV block? If so- which type?*

> <u>HINT</u>- Don't forget to consider *the most common cause of a pause* when formulating your answer.

Lead V$_1$

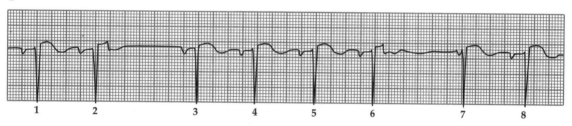

<u>Beyond the Core</u> → Note in the above rhythm that the PR interval of beat #7 is *shorter* than the PR interval of other conducted beats. *Why might this be* ?

Interpretation:

Applying the **4 Question Approach** to the rhythm that appears on page 287- we note the following:

    i) P waves *are* present. However, the atrial rate is *not* regular.

    ii) The QRS complex is *narrow* (i.e., *not* more than *half* a large box in duration).

    iii) The ventricular rhythm is *not* regular.

    iv) A relationship *does* exist between P waves and most QRS complexes- in the form of a *fixed* PR interval. This suggests that the *underlying* rhythm is **sinus**.

Comment → The rhythm on page 287 is a difficult tracing to interpret. At first glance- there appears to be *group beating*. Although recognition of group beating should always suggest the *possibility* of a Wenckebach-type conduction disorder- it is important to realize that *other* conditions may *also* produce this phenomenon. As emphasized on pages 273-274- the *most common cause* of a pause is a **blocked PAC**. This is the cause of the pause in this tracing. As noted above- the *underlying* rhythm is sinus. Careful inspection of the T waves at the *onset* of each pause (i.e., the T waves of beats #2 and 6)- reveals telltale *notching* of the blocked PAC (compared to the completely *smooth* T wave of other beats).

    Despite group beating- AV Wenckebach is *not* present in this tracing because the atrial rate is not regular and the PR interval does not prolong.

Beyond the Core → The PR interval that precedes beat #7 is *too short* to conduct. This implies that beat #7 must be a *junctional escape beat* that occurs *before* the P wave preceding it is able to conduct to the ventricles.

Review: *Is there AV block ?*

Use the **4 Question Approach** to interpret the rhythm shown below. *Is there AV block? If so- which type?*

> HINT- This rhythm was obtained from a completely healthy and playful young child.

Lead II

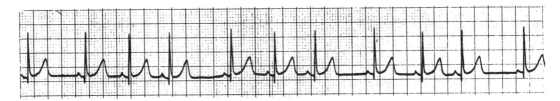

Additional Question → Why is this rhythm *not* Wenckebach?

Interpretation:

Applying the **4 Question Approach** to the rhythm that appears on page 289- we note the following:

i) & ii) The QRS complex is *narrow* (i.e., *not* more than *half* a large box in duration). The ventricular rhythm is *not* regular- although there *does* appear to be a *pattern* to the rhythm (i.e., there is *group beating*).

iii) P waves *are* present throughout the tracing. However- the atrial rhythm is clearly *not* regular.

iv) P waves *are* related to neighboring QRS complexes. Focusing on *each* QRS complex in the tracing- it can be seen that a P wave immediately *precedes* each QRS- and that the PR interval of this preceding P wave is constant. This suggests that each P wave *is* conducted- and that the mechanism of the rhythm must therefore be *sinus*. The reason for variability in the ventricular response is that the rhythm is **sinus arrhythmia**.

> **Comment** → Despite the presence of group beating- the rhythm that appears on page 289 does *not* represent AV Wenckebach. The other *KEY* footprints are absent. That is- the atrial rate is *not* regular, and the PR interval does *not* prolong with successive beats.
>
> The first clue to interpretation of this rhythm lies with the *history*- since we are told that the patient is an otherwise healthy and playful young child. AV block or other conduction disturbance would *not* be expected in this clinical setting. On the other hand (as emphasized on page 274)- **sinus arrhythmia** is a common *normal* finding in healthy children and young adults (in whom heart rate *often* varies in cyclical fashion with the pattern of respiration).

<u>Review</u>: *Is there AV block ?*

Use the **4 *Question Approach*** to interpret the rhythm shown below. *Is there AV block?* If so- *which type?*

> <u>HINT</u>- Be sure you have looked at the *entire* tracing before commenting on the presence (or absence) of atrial activity. *Do P waves ever have a chance to conduct ?*

Lead II

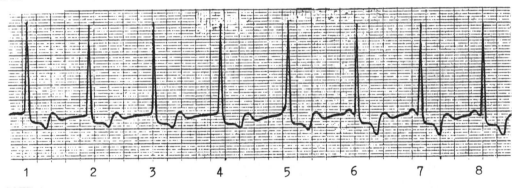

<u>Additional Question</u> → Should this patient be treated with cardiac pacing?

Interpretation:

Applying the **4 Question Approach** to the rhythm that appears on page 291- we note the following:

> i) & ii) The QRS complex is *narrow* (i.e., *not* more than *half* a large box in duration). The ventricular rhythm appears to vary slightly- although for the most part it is fairly regular (at a rate of 65-70 beats/minute).

> iii) & iv) P waves are *not* initially seen on this tracing. However- they clearly emerge during the latter part of the tracing (i.e., in front of beats #6, 7, and 8). A P wave also appears to be present in front of beat #5- *deforming* the upstroke of this complex. The PR interval for all of these beats appears short- and it is *definitely* too short to conduct in front of beat #5. Thus at least for a period of time, P waves are *unrelated* to QRS complexes- which defines the presence of **AV dissociation**.

> **Comment** → The rhythm that appears on page 291 is *not* a simple tracing. Yet interpretation is forthcoming with application of the systematic *4 Question Approach.* The initial 4 beats on the tracing represent a **junctional rhythm** (since the QRS complex is narrow, the ventricular rhythm fairly regular, and atrial activity is absent). The rate of 65-70 beats/minute makes this an **accelerated** junctional rhythm. Thereafter there is transient **AV dissociation**- since P waves are at least *temporarily* unrelated to QRS complexes. AV dissociation in this case is most likely the result of **usurpation** (*See* page 254)- from acceleration of the AV nodal pacemaker (to ≈70 beats/minute)- until finally toward the end of the tracing when P waves once again emerge.

KEY → There is absolutely *no evidence* of AV block on this tracing- because the P waves that are present *never* have a chance to conduct. Clinically- it is unlikely that pacemaker therapy will be needed as long as the ventricular rate remains adequate (and the patient remains hemodynamically stable).

<u>Review</u>: *Is there AV block ?*

Use the ***4 Question Approach*** to interpret the rhythm shown below. *Is there AV block?* If so- *which type?*

> <u>HINT</u>- Do P waves have a chance to conduct- *yet still fail to do so* ?

Lead II

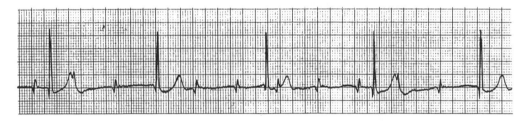

<u>Additional Questions:</u>

1. What *anatomic level* would you expect is the site of the block for the above tracing?

   > <u>HINT</u>- Consider QRS duration and the ventricular rate in formulating your response.

2. Is this patient likely to need cardiac pacing?

Interpretation:

Applying the **4 *Question Approach*** to the rhythm that appears on page 293- we note the following:

i) & ii) The QRS complex appears to be *narrow* (i.e., *not* more than *half* a large box in duration). The ventricular rhythm is *regular* and slow- with an R-R interval of just under 9 large boxes in duration (which corresponds to a ventricular rate of about 34 beats/minute).

iii) P waves *are* present throughout the tracing (albeit some of the P waves are *hidden* within QRS complexes). The atrial rhythm is regular- with a P-P interval of just over 3 large boxes in duration (which corresponds to an *atrial* rate of about 85-90/minute).

iv) P waves and neighboring QRS complexes are completely *unrelated*- as evidenced by the fact that the PR interval preceding each QRS complex *continually* changes (i.e., P waves "march through the QRS"). Thus, there is **complete AV dissociation** on this tracing.

> <u>**Comment**</u> → As opposed to the tracing on page 291 (in which P waves were *never* given adequate opportunity to conduct)- P waves in the tracing on page 293 are seen to occur at virtually *all* points in the cardiac cycle. Despite this- P waves *still* fail to conduct. Thus- *all* of the criteria listed on page 249 for diagnosis of **3° (complete) AV block** are met, including: 1) regular *atrial* rate; 2) regular *ventricular* rate; 3) *complete* AV dissociation; and 4) a sufficiently *slow* ventricular rate (i.e., ≤45 beats/minute)- so as to ensure adequate *opportunity* for normal conduction to occur.

<u>**Note**</u> → The presence of a narrow QRS complex suggests that the site of the block on page 293 originates from somewhere *within* the conduction system- most probably from the bundle of His given the *slow* ventricular rate *(See pages 219-220)*. Cardiac pacing is likely to be needed, since AV block is complete and the escape rate is so slow.

Section 2A- *Selected Advanced Concepts*

<u>Digitalis Toxicity</u>

Digitalis toxicity remains one of the most common *iatrogenic* illnesses that results in admission to the hospital. Although anorexia and nausea are often the first clinical signs- at times cardiac arrhythmias may be the *only* manifestation.

Clinically- digitalis is used in the treatment of congestive heart failure (as a positive inotropic agent)- and in the treatment of supraventricular tachyarrhythmias (especially rapid atrial fibrillation). The *therapeutic* effect of digitalis when used in the treatment of arrhythmias is primarily a result of its rate-slowing (i.e., *vagotonic*) action on the AV node. Unfortunately, there is a very narrow *"therapeutic window"* between doses of drug that are beneficial- and doses that lead to **digitalis toxicity**.

Adverse *arrhythmogenic effects* that are commonly seen with excessive digitalis include one or more of the following:

- excessive rate slowing
- manifestations of various forms of heart block
- acceleration of subsidiary (i.e., *escape*) pacemakers
- enhanced automaticity of ectopic foci (in the atria, AV node,
      and ventricles)

Question → Which arrhythmias would you expect to see most commonly with digitalis toxicity?

<u>HINT</u>- Consider the above *arrhythmogenic* effects of the drug in formulating your answer.

Cardiac Arrhythmias and Digitalis Toxicity

Practically speaking- digitalis toxicity can produce virtually *any* cardiac arrhythmia (except perhaps atrial flutter and *rapid* atrial fibrillation). There are however, certain arrhythmias that are particularly characteristic of digitalis toxicity- such that their recognition should routinely suggest the *possibility* of this diagnosis *whenever* these arrhythmias are seen in a patient who is taking the drug. These arrhythmias include:

- inappropriate (and excessive) sinus bradycardia and/or arrhythmia
- sinus pauses or sinus arrest
- sinoatrial (SA) block
- 1° AV block
- 2° AV block, Mobitz type I (Wenckebach)
- *Wenckebach-type* conduction with atrial flutter or fibrillation
- atrial tachycardia with block
- atrial fibrillation when the ventricular response is very *slow*- or when there is *regularization* of the ventricular response
- *accelerated* junctional escape rhythms (or junctional tachycardia)
- increased ventricular ectopy- especially in the form of ventricular bigeminy, frequent multiform PVCs, or ventricular tachycardia.

> **Note** → Be especially alert to the *possibility* of digitalis toxicity in the setting of clinical situations that *predispose* to its development. These include the presence of impaired renal function (since the drug is primarily excreted by the kidneys), hypoxemia, hypokalemia, hypomagnesemia, and acute myocardial infarction. Lower maintenance doses are generally recommended in the elderly (i.e., 0.125 mg per day or less- instead of the usual 0.25 mg daily dose)- since older patients are particularly prone to developing digitalis toxicity (especially if renal function is already somewhat impaired).

Problem: *How to Approach this Rhythm ?*

The tracing shown below was obtained from an elderly woman with syncopal episodes and a history of heart failure.

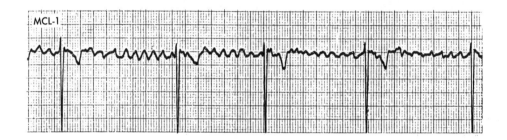

Questions:

1. How would you interpret this rhythm?

2. What *two* clinical conditions are most likely to produce this arrhythmia?

> HINT- Referral to pages 295-296 suggests one of the answers. The other condition is the most common cause of bradyarrhythmias in an elderly patient.

3. What *historical* information would you want most to obtain from this patient?

Answer:

The rhythm that appears on page 297 is *irregularly* irregular- and the ventricular response is extremely *slow* (i.e., between 35-50 beats/minute). Definite P waves are absent. Instead there are coarse undulations in the baseline that have the appearance of "fib waves" (as described on page 105-106). We therefore interpret this rhythm as **atrial fibrillation (A Fib)**- with an extremely **slow ventricular response**.

As noted on page 107- new-onset A Fib is most often accompanied by a *rapid* ventricular response. When the heart rate is uncharacteristically slow (as it is on page 297)- several predisposing conditions should be considered:

    i) *Digitalis toxicity.*
    ii) Use of *another* potentially rate-slowing agent (such as verapamil, diltiazem, and/or a
        beta-blocker).
    iii) *Sick sinus syndrome (SSS).*

Use of Digoxin is common in patients with a history of heart failure (as this patient had). Because renal function declines with age, elderly individuals are especially predisposed to development of digitalis toxicity. Other antiarrhythmic agents (as listed above) might also produce excessive slowing of the ventricular response to A Fib. Historically then, obtaining a complete list of this patient's *medications* would be essential to formulating an optimal approach to her care (since *withdrawal* of one or more drugs might be all that is needed if the bradycardia was drug-induced).

Practically speaking- if this patient was *not* toxic from digitalis- and she was *not* on other potentially rate-slowing medication)- then the *most likely* explanation for her excessive bradycardia would be **Sick Sinus Syndrome (SSS)**. Cardiac pacing might then be the treatment of choice for her syncopal episodes.

> **Note →** Clinical manifestations of SSS are discussed in detail on pages 303-304. The point to emphasize here is that the diagnosis of SSS should *never* be made until *iatrogenic* causes (i.e., excessive use of rate-slowing drugs) has been considered and ruled out.

Problem: *How to Approach this Rhythm ?*

The tracing shown below was obtained from a patient who was being treated for rapid atrial fibrillation with Digoxin. *How would you interpret this rhythm ?*

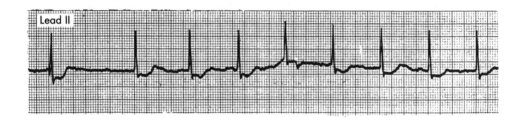

Additional Questions:

1. If told that this patient was *still* in A Fib- how might you explain the surprisingly *regular* ventricular response?

HINT- Feel free to refer to page 296 in formulating your answer.

2. How would you treat this patient?

Answer:

The most helpful clue to interpreting the rhythm that appears on page 299 lies with the clinical history- which tells us that the patient has been in atrial fibrillation- and was being treated with Digoxin.

After the first two beats in the tracing- the rhythm becomes surprisingly *regular*. The QRS complex is *narrow* (i.e., *not* more than *half* a large box in duration). Although there are fine undulations in the baseline- definite P waves are *not* seen in this lead II monitoring lead. Therefore, the rhythm *can't* be of sinus origin.

This patient is actually *still* in A Fib! The reason for "*regularization*" of the ventricular response is a direct result of **digitalis toxicity**. As noted on page 296- digitalis toxicity may produce many different types of cardiac arrhythmias. The mechanism responsible for the phenomenon of **regularization** of A Fib is complete (or at least *almost* complete) AV block from digitalis toxicity- with resultant *escape* of a regular and slightly *accelerated* junctional pacemaker (shown here at a rate of about 75 beats/minute).

Treatment of this rhythm is simple- *withdrawal* of digitalis. As the serum level of the drug decreases, ECG abnormalities should resolve- so that the irregularly irregular rhythm of this patient's underlying A Fib should once again be seen. If continued use of Digoxin was still needed, a lower maintenance dose of drug might then be advisable.

> **Note** → Regularization of A Fib and accelerated junctional rhythms are highly suggestive clues to the presence of digitalis toxicity. This diagnosis should be suspected *whenever* either of these rhythms is seen in a patient taking the drug.

Problem: *How to Approach this Rhythm ?*

The tracing shown below was obtained from a patient who was being treated with Digoxin for congestive heart failure. The patient had been in normal sinus rhythm (NSR). *How would you interpret this rhythm ?*

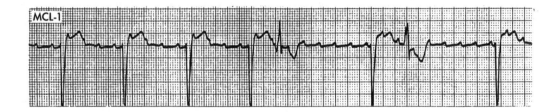

Additional Questions:

1. Is the patient still in NSR? (Are *any* P waves conducting?)

2. Can you think of a single *unifying* diagnosis to account for *all* of the abnormal findings that are seen on this tracing?

> HINT- Feel free to again refer to page 296 in formulating your answer.

Answer:

The underlying rhythm for the tracing that appears on page 301 is **atrial tachycardia**. The atrial rate is regular and extremely rapid- with a P-P interval that is slightly over one large box in duration. By the *'Every OTHER Beat' Method* (See pages 55-58)- we estimate the atrial rate to be about **220 beats/minute**.

Two types of QRS complexes are seen on this tracing. The more commonly occurring form has an rS configuration- and is seen for the first four beats on the tracing. The QRS complex for these first four beats does *not* appear to be widened (i.e., it is *not more* than half a large box in duration). Note that a P wave precedes each of these four beats with a *fixed* PR interval- suggesting that these beats *are* being conducted. However, many more P waves are *not* being conducted- as evidenced by shortening of the PR interval later on in the tracing and the presence of numerous P waves that are *not* followed by a QRS complex. Thus, there is evidence of **AV block** which looks to be severe (i.e., *high grade-* or *high degree*) given the number of P waves that fail to conduct.

The last finding on this tracing relates to the two beats that manifest a predominantly upright (qRs and Rs) configuration. Both of these beats are presumably **PVCs**- given their early occurrence, different morphology, and QRS widening.

As suggested on page 296- the *combination* of findings described above (i.e. atrial tachycardia- high grade AV block- and PVCs)- is highly suggestive of **digitalis toxicity**.

> **KEY** → This is a difficult tracing! We emphasize that some of the subtleties described above clearly extend *beyond* the scope of this book. Nevertheless- consider your interpretation accurate if you recognized the atrial tachycardia- the presence of at least *some* degree of AV block- and the PVCs. In turn, we consider our objective accomplished if we have succeeded in increasing your index of suspicion for detecting *digitalis toxicity* in patients who are taking this drug- and who present with one or more of the arrhythmias listed on page 296.

Sick Sinus Syndrome

Sick Sinus Syndrome (SSS) is a commonly encountered entity among the elderly. The syndrome encompasses a wide variety of cardiac arrhythmias that can most easily be recalled by reflecting on its name (i.e., *"sick sinus"*)- which alludes to the progressive *deterioration* that occurs in sinus node function. One might therefore expect to see one or more of the following arrhythmias:

- persistent *sinus bradycardia* (which is the most common and often
  the earliest manifestation of SSS)
- sinus *arrhythmia*- which may be marked and is often seen with
  sinus bradycardia
- sinus *pauses*- which may be frequent and become progressively more
  prolonged (and eventually lead to *sinus arrest*)
- SA (sinoatrial) block- in which exit block *out of* the sinus node results in
  failure of some sinus impulses to be transmitted to the atria
- atrial fibrillation with a *slow* ventricular response.

There are two additional commonly seen components to SSS:

1) <u>*Associated AV nodal disease*</u>- reflecting the fact that most patients with SSS also have a *"sick"* AV node. As a result, escape rhythms with SSS tend to be *slow*- be this in the form of *slow* A Fib (as seen on page 297)- or in the form of a *slow* junctional escape rhythm.

2) <u>*Tachy rhythms*</u>- reflecting the other extreme of a malfunctioning sinus node- in which *rapid* rhythms (most commonly *rapid* atrial fibrillation or flutter, PSVT, or atrial tachycardia) are seen in many (but *not* all) patients with SSS (hence its alternate name, ***"Tachy-Brady" Syndrome***).

Question → How is the diagnosis of SSS made clinically? How should patients with SSS be treated (if they should be treated)?

Sick Sinus Syndrome

The diagnosis of SSS is made clinically by recognition of one or more of the arrhythmias that are listed on page 303- *when* they occur in the appropriate clinical setting. As might be imagined, development of SSS is often an insidious process that occurs over a number of *years*-which is why many patients are *unaware* that they have (or are developing) the syndrome. As a result, SSS often goes *undiagnosed* for long periods of time- especially when the subject is an elderly individual who is *not* very active- and whose major manifestation of SSS is sinus brady-cardia *without* long pauses.

In contrast, the diagnosis of SSS is much more likely to be made sooner when the arrhythmias it produces result in significant symptoms. As might be imagined, common clinical manifestations of SSS are syncope or presyncope (from prolonged sinus pauses or sinus arrest)- and weakness or congestive heart failure (from persistent and severe bradycardia- with an *inability* to appropriately increase heart rate in response to activity). Other patients present with symptoms from tachyarrhythmias (i.e., palpitations from rapid A Fib).

As emphasized on pages 297-298- a *KEY* aspect of diagnosis is to *rule out* the possibility of an *iatrogenic* cause of the patient's arrhythmias (most commonly from digitalis toxicity or *other* rate-slowing drugs). Other potential causes of severe bradycardia should be actively considered (i.e., myocardial infarction, hypothyroidism, electrolyte disorders, etc).

Treatment of SSS → is completely dependent on the nature and severity of the patient's symptoms. Pacemaker implantation is indicated for **symptomatic bradycardia** that is not the result of an acute process (such as Acute MI or drug toxicity). In contrast, the elderly subject who is completely *asymptomatic* from SSS- may *not* be in need of any treatment at all.

Medication is generally recommended for initial treatment of tachyarrhythmias- with the problem being that use of rate-slowing drugs will often only control the *tachy* part of the *Tachy-Brady Syndrome*- at the expense of exacerbating the severity of the brady-cardia. Cardiac pacing- *as well as* rate-slowing medication- may be needed for treatment of such patients.

Problem: *How to Approach this Rhythm ?*

The tracings shown below were obtained from an elderly patient with syncope. *How would you interpret these rhythms ?*

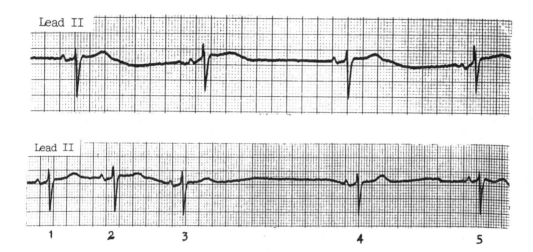

Additional Question → What clinical considerations should be in your differential diagnosis? What treatment is indicated?

Answer:

The *TOP* rhythm that appears on page 305 is slow and slightly irregular. We estimate the heart rate to be about 35 beats/minute (since the R-R interval is between 8 and 9 large boxes in duration). The QRS complex is *not* widened (since the QRS is *not more* than half a large box in duration). P waves *are* present- and can be seen to precede each QRS complex with a *fixed* PR interval. The mechanism of this rhythm is therefore *sinus*- and we interpret the tracing as showing **sinus bradycardia** and **arrhythmia**. Note that the PR interval is *not more* than a large box in duration- which means that it is still within the normal range.

The *LOWER* tracing on page 305 begins as **sinus rhythm** (at a rate of 60 beats/minute) for the first 3 beats on the tracing. Thereafter follows a long *pause* before each of the next two beats. Despite these pauses- the QRS complex remains narrow and virtually identical in morphology to the QRS complexes of beats #1-3. Sinus P waves with a constant PR interval precede all 5 beats on the tracing. Thus, the basic mechanism is still sinus- in this case with two **sinus pauses** (that occur after beats #3 and #4). Note that the pause following beat #3 is *over* 2.6 seconds (i.e., more than 13 large boxes) in duration.

Comment → Taken together, the findings present on these two tracings (i.e., sinus bradycardia and arrhythmia- and prolonged sinus pauses)- in conjunction with the history (i.e., syncope in an elderly patient)- are highly suggestive of **Sick Sinus Syndrome**. Assuming the absence of a potentially reversible cause of these arrhythmias (i.e., drug toxicity, acute MI, hypothyroidism, electrolyte disturbance, etc.)- cardiac *pacing* is likely to be needed.

Problem: *How to Approach this Rhythm ?*

The irregularly irregular rhythm shown below was obtained from a middle-aged man with a history of COPD (chronic obstructive pulmonary disease). Why is this *not* atrial fibrillation?

>   HINT- Are P waves present? If so- does it look like the P waves are origi-
>   nating from the same site in the atria?

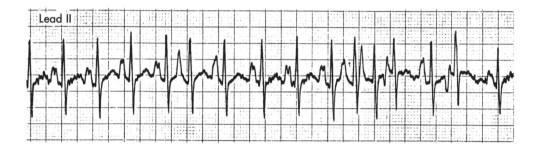

Additional Question → Why is it important to distinguish
  between atrial fibrillation and the cause of the irregularly irregular
  rhythm shown above?

Answer:

Despite the fact that the rhythm on page 307 is *irregularly* irregular- this is *not* A Fib. We say this because definite P waves *are* present throughout the tracing. Although most P waves are positive (with either a pointed or notched configuration)- some are biphasic. Overall, P wave morphology *continually* changes- and no predominant form is noted. This suggests that P waves arise from multiple *different* sites in the atria. We therefore interpret the rhythm as **MAT** (**M**ultifocal **A**trial **T**achycardia).

As alluded to on pages 109-110- the importance of distinguishing between rapid A Fib and MAT is that the clinical course and treatment of these two arrhythmias is very different. Rapid atrial fibrillation is the much more common disorder- occurring in many types of patients (especially the elderly). In the acute setting *digitalization* constitutes a medical treatment of choice. Many clinicians use the rapidity of the ventricular response as a way to gauge the amount of IV digoxin to administer.

In contrast- MAT occurs primarily in two clinical settings: 1) in patients with COPD; and 2) in severely ill patients with multisystem disease. Treatment of MAT *must* be directed at correcting the *underlying* cause of the arrhythmia- which usually entails correction of hypoxemia, acidosis, electrolyte abnormalties, and other systemic illness. The clinical point to emphasize is that MAT is notoriously *resistant* to treatment with digoxin- and that these patients are extremely susceptible to developing digitalis toxicity.

KEY → The *KEY* to diagnosing MAT is to maintain a high index of suspicion for this disorder in the clinical settings in which it is most likely to occur (i.e., in patients with severe pulmonary disease and acutely ill ICU patients). Be aware that this irregularly irregular rhythm may simulate A Fib if P waves are not well seen in the lead being monitored- so that if doubt exists- *additional* leads (and *ideally* a 12-lead ECG) should be obtained to clarify the nature of atrial activity.

Problem: *How to Approach this Rhythm ?*

The tracing shown below was obtained from a middle-aged adult on digoxin. The patient had been in sinus rhythm. *What is going on* ?

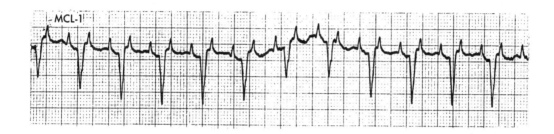

Additional Questions:

1. Is the rhythm shown above more likely to be *atrial flutter-* or *atrial tachycardia* with block?

> HINT- Consider the *atrial* rate and the *clinical scenario* in formulating your answer.

2. What are the clinical implications of the above rhythm?

Answer:

The rhythm that appears on page 309 is *regular* at a rate of about 115 beats/minute. P waves *are* present- and outnumber QRS complexes by two to one- making the atrial rate about 230/minute. The QRS complex is *narrow* (implying a *supraventricular* mechanism)- and each QRS complex *is* preceded by a P wave with a constant PR interval. Thus, P waves *are* related to the QRS complexes- albeit only one out of every two P waves is being conducted to the ventricles. We interpret this rhythm as ***atrial tachycardia*** *with* **2:1 AV block**.

Comment → This is a difficult tracing! The diagnostic dilemma it illustrates is having to distinguish between atrial flutter with 2:1 AV conduction- and atrial tachycardia with 2:1 AV block. There are several reasons why we favor the latter diagnosis in this case. The first relates to the heart rate. As emphasized on page 112- the atrial rate of flutter is almost always *close* to 300 beats/minute (usual range = 250-350/minute)- *unless* the patient is being treated with a drug such as quinidine, procainamide, verapamil, or diltiazem which may slow the atrial rate. Digoxin does *not* slow the atrial rate of flutter. In addition, the typical *sawtooth* pattern of atrial flutter is absent. Instead, the baseline between P waves is flat (i.e., *isoelectric*).

The final reason we favor the diagnosis of atrial tachycardia with block is the clinical scenario (i.e., the fact that the patient had been in sinus rhythm and was being treated with digoxin. Although it is possible that atrial flutter could have suddenly developed- a much more likely scenario is that there is now digitalis toxicity. As emphasized on page 296- atrial tachycardia with block is a characteristic manifestation of digitalis toxicity- and this diagnosis should *always* be suspected *whenever* this rhythm is seen in a patient who is taking digoxin.

Problem: *How to Approach this Rhythm ?*

The tracing shown below was obtained from a middle-aged woman with new-onset palpitations. The patient was alert and hemodynamically stable at the time the rhythm was recorded. The tracing was interpreted as showing *atrial fibrillation* with a rapid ventricular response. *Do you agree* ?

Lead II

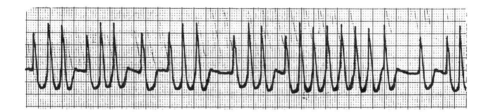

Additional Questions:

1. What is distinctly unusual about this example of atrial fibrillation?

HINT- How fast is the rhythm at its most rapid point?

2. Why is this *unlikely* to be ventricular tachycardia?

Answer:

The rhythm that appears on page 311 is extremely rapid and irregularly irregular. No atrial activity is seen in this lead II recording. Although the QRS complex is definitely widened- the gross irregularity of this rhythm makes VT unlikely. This leaves **atrial fibrillation** as the most probable diagnosis.

The thing that is most unusual about this example of A Fib is the rate. Under normal conditions with A Fib, the refractory period of the AV node does *not* allow more than 150-200 impulses per minute to be conducted to the ventricles. The ventricular response is clearly faster than this in certain parts of this tracing. In such places, the R-R interval is just over one large box in duration- which corresponds to a heart rate of about **250 beats/minute**. This is far *too fast* for atrial impulses to be transmitted over the normal (AV nodal) conduction pathway. The most logical explanation is that atrial impulses must be *bypassing* the AV node- and are being conducted to the ventricles via an **accessory pathway (AP)** with a much shorter refractory period. The patient must therefore have **WPW** (i.e., **W**olff-**P**arkinson-**W**hite) syndrome.

KEY → WPW is a syndrome in which one or more *accessory* conduction pathways exist that allow an alternate route for transmission of the electrical impulse from the atria to the ventricles. The incidence of this syndrome is approximately 2 cases per 1,000 in the general population. **WPW** is recognized on a 12-lead ECG by the presence of PR interval shortening- slurring of the initial upstroke of the QRS complex (the **delta wave**)- and QRS widening. It should be suspected *whenever* A Fib is seen at an exceedingly rapid rate (i.e., >220/minute)- as is the case on page 311.

Clinically- the importance of recognizing WPW (and distinguishing it from "ordinary" A Fib)- is that treatment with digoxin, verapamil, and/or diltiazem is *contraindicated* (because each of these drugs may further *accelerate* antegrade conduction down the AP). The treatment of choice for WPW with rapid A Fib is **IV procainamide** (which *slows* antegrade conduction down the AP)- and/or synchronized cardioversion.

<u>Problem:</u> *How to Approach this Rhythm* ?

The tracing shown below was recorded from a patient who had overdosed on an unknown medication. The patient was unresponsive- so that no additional history was obtainable. *How would you interpret this rhythm* ?

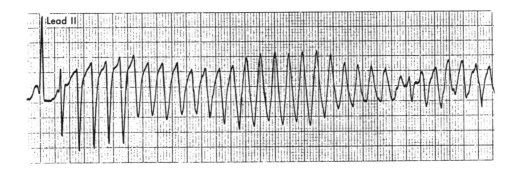

<u>Additional Questions:</u>

1. Why is this rhythm *not* simply ventricular tachycardia?

> <u>HINT</u>- What happens to QRS morphology during the tracing?

2. How should the patient be treated?

Answer:

The very first beat on the tracing shown on page 313 is narrow and upright. This is presumably a *supraventricular* impulse- although admittedly, additional rhythm strips would be needed to verify this presumption. Thereafter, the rhythm changes dramatically. That is- the QRS complex *widens*- and a "slinky"-like configuration of *alternating polarity* (first negative- then positive- then negative again toward the end of the tracing) is seen. This pattern is characteristic of **Torsade de Pointes**.

KEY → The term *Torsade de Pointes* was first described by the French physician Dessertene in 1966- and literally means- *"twisting of the points"*. The rhythm is all too often incorrectly diagnosed as "ordinary" ventricular tachycardia (or ventricular fibrillation). This can be a potentially *lethal* mistake if the incorrect treatment is given.

Torsade is frequently associated with a long QT interval on the baseline ECG. The arrhythmia is thought to be triggered by the occurrence of a PVC at a relatively late point during the repolarization process. Paroxysms of wide complex tachycardia with *alternating polarity* ensue (which distinguish this rhythm from "ordinary" VT). These paroxysms often terminate spontaneously- but frequently recur until the underlying predisposing cause of QT prolongation has been corrected.

The most important causes of Torsade are those conditions that produce QT prolongation- especially Type IA antiarrhythmic agents (i.e., quinidine, procainamide)- phenothiazine or tricyclic antidepressant overdose- and/or hypokalemia/hypomagnesemia.

The treatment of choice for Torsade is **magnesium sulfate** (often in large doses of 2-5 g IV- or more). Overdrive pacing is sometimes used. The precipitating agents must be withdrawn- and antiarrhythmic agents such as procainamide (that may further lengthen the QT interval) must be avoided.

Aberrant Conduction

- *Definition/Diagnostic Criteria* -

One of the most difficult problems confronting those involved in emergency cardiac care is the differentiation of PVCs from PACs (or PJCs) that are conducted with *aberration*. Consider the following example. If told that the tracing shown below was obtained from a patient with acute myocardial infarction:

1. Would you interpret the rhythm as sinus with frequent PVCs (including a ventricular couplet toward the end of the tracing)- and *therefore* treat the patient with lidocaine?   - *or* -

2. Would you interpret the abnormal-looking beats as PACs that are *aberrantly* conducted- and therefore *not* treat with antiarrhythmic drugs?

Lead MCL1

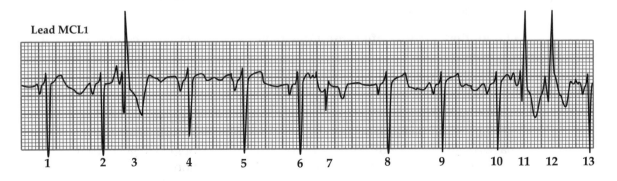

Aberrant Conduction

Definition→ QRS widening that results from conduction of premature *supraventricular* impulses (PACs or PJCs) that occur at a time when a portion of the conduction system is still refractory.

Importance → PVCs that are *new* in onset- especially if frequent and *repetitive* (i.e., occurring in couplets, salvos, or longer runs of ventricular tachycardia)- should probably be treated when they occur in the setting of acute ischemic heart disease (i.e., unstable angina- or Acute MI). IV lidocaine is the usual drug of choice.

In contrast- *aberrantly* conducted PACs (or PJCs) should *not* be treated with lidocaine, since use of this drug is *not* completely benign. Hence the importance of distinguishing between PVCs and aberrantly conducted beats is that the former may need to be treated (if the setting is *acute* ischemic heart disease)- and the latter does not.

Diagnostic Criteria → The most helpful criteria for determining if abnormal looking (i.e., *anomalous*) beats are PVCs or aberrantly conducted are:

i) The presence of a *typical* **R**ight **B**undle **B**ranch **B**lock (**RBBB**) pattern for the anomalous complex when viewed from a *right-sided* monitoring lead (i.e., lead V_1 or MCL_1).

ii) A **similar *initial* deflection** for anomalous and normally conducted beats.

iii) The finding of a ***premature* P wave** before the anomalous beat.

iv) A ***"reason"*** for aberrant conduction to occur.

As we explain on the next few pages- these diagnostic criteria are *all* present for *each* of the abnormal beats in the rhythm shown on page 315 (i.e., for beats #3, 7, 11, and 12). This strongly suggests that all of these beats are PACs conducted with aberration.

Aberrant Conduction

- *A Closer Look at the Features* -

Examine the tracing below which magnifies the first 5 beats from the rhythm strip shown on page 315. Is the third beat a PVC- or a PAC conducted with *aberration*?

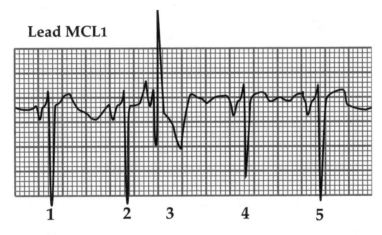

Lead MCL1

Additional Questions:

1. Which of the diagnostic criteria for *aberrant* conduction that we listed on page 316 are seen above?

2. With what *degree of certainty* do you place in your answer?

Answer:

One can say with *almost* **100% certainty**- that the third beat in this tracing is a **PAC** (for which the QRS complex is widened because of **aberrant** conduction. All of the diagnostic criteria listed on page 316 are met:

i) The anomalous complex manifests a **typical RBBB pattern** in this *right-sided* monitoring lead (*See Comment below*).

ii) A **similar *initial* deflection** is seen for the third beat (which is *upward* in the form of a tiny but *positive* r wave)- as for the slightly larger r waves that comprise the initial deflection of the normally conducted beats.

iii) The anomalous beat is preceded by a **premature P wave**- seen here as producing the extra *peaking* in the T wave that immediately precedes the widened beat.

iv) A definite **"reason"** for aberrant conduction exists. That is- the third beat in this tracing occurs at a sufficiently early point in the cardiac cycle that one might *reasonably* expect a portion of the conduction system (in this case- the *right* bundle branch)- to still be in a refractory state.

Comment → We first introduced the system for *QRS Nomenclature* on pages 29-38. One of the most important clinical applications of this system relates to its use for assessing QRS morphology of anomalous complexes in the differentiation of PVCs from aberrancy. Aberrant beats most often conduct with a pattern of RBBB. In a **typical RBBB pattern**- an rsR' (or rSR' or RSR') complex is seen in a *right-sided* monitoring lead (i.e., V_1 or MCL_1)- in which the S wave must *at least* descend to the baseline- and the *second* R wave peak (the R') must be *taller* than the initial r wave (so as to produce a **"taller right rabbit ear"**). These morphologic characteristics are all well seen in the third beat shown on page 317. Together with the other criteria noted above, we can be virtually 100% certain that the reason for QRS widening of this beat is aberrant conduction.

A *"Reason"* for Aberrancy

As we have emphasized- an important criterion for determining if an anomalous complex is aberrant or not is that there should be a *"reason"* for aberrant conduction to occur. That is- the anomalous complex should occur sufficiently *early* in the cycle- such that a portion of the conduction system is still likely to be refractory.

Apply this concept to the tracing shown below. Would you expect beat #4 to be a PVC- or a PAC conducted with aberration?

>HINT- **Always assume that a beat is *"guilty"* (i.e.,** *ventricular* in origin)-
>**until** *proven* **"innocent" (i.e.,** *aberrantly* conducted).

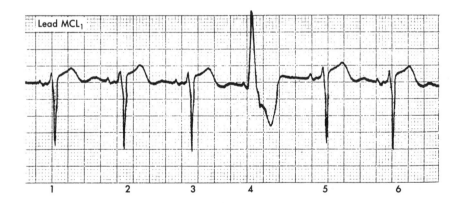

Additional Question → Note that a P wave *does* precede beat #4!
Is this P wave premature ? (Does the *timing* of this P wave provide an additional clue to the etiology of beat #4?)

Answer:

The *underlying* rhythm that appears on page 319 is **sinus**- with the *exception* of beat #4. Other than this slightly early and very *different* appearing beat- the underlying ventricular rhythm is regular with an R-R interval of just over 4 large boxes in duration (corresponding to a rate of just under 75 beats/minute). Note that each sinus beat is preceded by a P wave with a constant and normal PR interval. QRS duration of sinus-conducted beats is at the upper limit of normal (i.e., about *half* a large box in duration).

Beat #4 is *definitely* a **PVC**. This beat is wide and bizarre in appearance- with a *morphology* that is very suggestive of a ventricular etiology (i.e., it completely *lacks* the RBBB pattern of aberrant conduction described on pages 316 and 318).

Note that beat #4 *is* preceded by a P wave. However, this P wave is *not* premature! Instead, it occurs right *on time* with respect to the atrial rate for other P waves in this tracing (i.e., the atrial rate remains regular *throughout* the tracing). Note also that the PR interval preceding each sinus-conducted beat (i.e., the PR interval of beats #1-3, 5, and 6) is about 0.17 second in duration. The fact that the PR interval preceding beat #4 is much *shorter* than this means that adequate time did *not* exist for sinus conduction to occur (which here requires 0.17 second). Thus- *"something else"* must have occurred to produce the QRS complex of beat #4 *other than* a sinus beat- with the two possibilities being a PJC or a PVC.

We emphasized in the Clinical Note on page 158 that PJCs are relatively uncommon. Furthermore, PJCs are usually narrow and very similar in appearance to sinus conducted beats. Although the possibility that beat #4 is a PJC that somehow conducts with aberration can *not* be ruled out- this possibility would seem to be much less likely than our assumption that beat #4 is a ventricular beat (i.e., *assume a beat "guilty"- until proven otherwise*).

Final support of our assumption that beat #4 is a PVC is forthcoming from the fact that **there is simply *no reason* to expect aberrant conduction**. That is- beat #4 occurs so *late* with respect to the preceding T wave that the ventricular conduction system should have had more than enough time to completely recover. This is in marked contrast to the situation with the anomalous beats in the rhythm on page 315- which all occur at a much *earlier* point in the cardiac cycle.

The *Relative* Refractory Period

- *Why Some Beats Conduct Aberrantly* -

Examine the schematic Figure shown below.

1. Would you expect an *early* occurring *supraventricular* impulse (PAC or PJC) to be conducted if it arrives at the ventricles during the **ARP** (<u>**A**</u>bsolute <u>**R**</u>efractory <u>**P**</u>eriod)- indicated by point **A** in the Figure?

2. What if the early occurring impulse arrives during the **RRP** (<u>**R**</u>elative <u>**R**</u>efractory **P**eriod)- indicated by point **B** in the Figure? If the premature impulse *is* conducted to the ventricles- *would you expect such conduction to be normal* ?

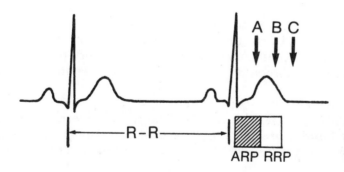

Answer:

Early occurring supraventricular impulses that arrive at the AV node may or may not be conducted on to the ventricles. The major determinant of whether or not such conduction takes place is the state of refractoriness of the ventricular conduction system at the time the electrical impulse arrives at the bundle of His. If the process of ventricular repolarization is complete at this time (and the ventricular conduction system has *fully* recovered)- then the electrical impulse will be conducted *normally* to the ventricles (and a narrow, normal appearing QRS complex will be seen). This should be the case for premature **impulse C** in the Figure that appears on page 321 (as well as for *any other* supraventricular impulse that occurs *later* in the cycle than impulse C).

On the other hand- if the premature impulse arrives too *early* in the repolarization process- it may find the ventricles *physiologically* unable to conduct the stimulus. This is the situation represented by premature **impulse A** in the Figure- which is seen to occur during the *absolute* refractory period (ARP). PACs or PJCs that occur during this period will be *"blocked"* (i.e., *not* conducted to the ventricles). Clinically (as emphasized on pages 160 and 274)- *the most common cause of a pause-* is a *blocked* PAC.

Aberrant conduction occurs when a premature impulse arrives at a moment in time that is *intermediate* to points A and C in the Figure. This situation is represented by premature **impulse B**- which is seen to occur during the *relative* refractory period (RRP). At this time in the repolarization process, a *portion* of the ventricular conduction system has recovered- *but another portion has not.*

Practically speaking- aberrant conduction manifests the pattern of *block* for that part of the conduction system that is late (last) to recover. The reason aberrantly conducted beats most often take on a **right bundle branch block (RBBB) pattern**- is that under normal circumstances, the refractory period of the right bundle branch tends to be *longer* than the refractory period of the other two major conduction fascicles. It should be emphasized, however, that aberrant conduction may *also* take on the form of a left bundle branch block (LBBB) pattern- or of either a LAHB (left *anterior* hemiblock) or LPHB (left *posterior* hemiblock) pattern- *or any combination thereof.*

<u>Problem:</u> *PVCs or Aberrant ?*

- *Why does beat #10 look so different?* -

Examine the tracing shown below. Is beat #10 a PVC? Why does this beat look *different* than beat #6? Can you explain the *pause* after beat #2?

> <u>HINT</u>- Feel free to refer to the Figure on page 321 in formulating your answers.

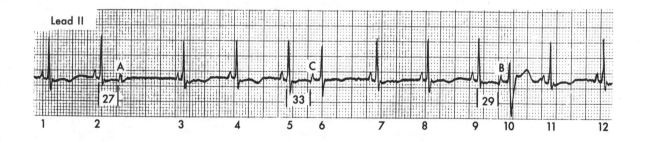

<u>Additional Question</u> → Can *QRS morphology* (i.e., the presence or absence of a RBBB pattern)- be used to help to determine if beat #10 is a PVC in the above tracing? If not- *why not* ?

Answer:

The *underlying* rhythm for the tracing that appears on page 323 is **sinus**. Premature atrial contractions (**PACs**) notch the T waves of beats #2, #5, and #9. The PAC that occurs *earliest* (labeled **A** in this Figure) is **blocked**. This premature impulse has the shortest *coupling* interval (0.27 second- as measured here from the onset of the R wave until the onset of the premature P wave)- and corresponds to the premature impulse labeled A on page 321 (which occurs during the ARP). Thus, the *cause* of the *pause* in the rhythm- is a *blocked* PAC.

Beats #6 and #10 in the rhythm are **aberrantly conducted**- with the latter complex manifesting a greater degree of aberrancy. This is because premature impulse **B** occurs at an *earlier* point (it has the shorter coupling interval of 0.29 second)- when the conduction system is more refractory (corresponding to premature impulse B on page 321). Premature impulse **C** has the longest coupling interval (of 0.33 second)- and probably occurs late in the RRP. As a result, beat #6 is conducted with only a minimal degree of aberration. Were this PAC to occur any later, it would most likely fall beyond the refractory period and be conducted normally.

Note → Morphologic characteristics that were previously discussed relating to the presence of a *typical* RBBB pattern (rsR' configuration with taller *right* rabbit ear)- can *not* be applied to the rhythm on page 323- because a *right-sided* monitoring lead (V_1 or MCL_1) was *not* used !!!

Beyond the Core → It was emphasized on page 322 that although aberrantly conducted beats most often manifest a RBBB pattern (because the refractory period of the right bundle branch tends to be *longer* than that of the other major conduction fascicles)- aberrant conduction may also manifest *other* patterns of bundle branch block and/or hemiblock. This is illustrated by beat #10 on page 323 which conducts with a pattern of left *anterior* hemiblock (LAHB) aberration.

The *"Typical"* RBBB Pattern

- *QRS Morphology in Lead V₁ or MCL₁* -

Examine the schematic QRS complexes (labeled **A** through **H**) that appear in the Figure below. For which of these schematic complexes are conditions met to satisfy description as a ***"typical"* RBBB pattern** ?

> HINT- As emphasized on page 318- a *typical* RBBB pattern should manifest an rsR' (or rSR' or RSR')- with a **taller *right* rabbit ear**- *as well as* an S wave that descends *back down* to the baseline.

	Suggestive of a SUPRAVENTRICULAR Etiology/Aberration	Of NO HELP in Differentiation	Suggestive of a VENTRICULAR Etiology
Right-sided monitoring leads (such as V₁ or MCL₁)	Taller RIGHT rabbit ear — A B	Taller RIGHT rabbit ear — C D E	Taller LEFT rabbit ear — F G H

The "Typical" RBBB Pattern of Aberrant Conduction

For conditions of a "typical" RBBB pattern to be satisfied, there should be:

- an **rsR' pattern** (or *equivalent* configuration)

- in a **right-sided monitoring lead** (V_1 or MCL_1)

- with a **taller *right* rabbit ear**- and -

- an **S wave** that **descends** *back down* to the baseline.

These conditions are met for schematic complexes **A** and **B** that appear on page 325 (which manifest an RsR' and rsR' configuration, respectively- each with an S wave that descends *below* the baseline- and a taller *right* rabbit ear). Although admittedly *not* 100% diagnostic- the presence of a *typical* RBBB pattern in a *right-sided* monitoring lead (as seen for complexes A and B) greatly increases the likelihood that the beat in question is *aberrantly* conducted (and *supraventricular* in etiology).

In contrast- when the *left* rabbit ear is taller (i.e., when the initial positive deflection is taller than the second [R'] positive deflection)- then ventricular ectopy is strongly suggested (complex **F** in the Figure). A ventricular etiology is also suggested by an "R-slur-prime" configuration (complex **G**) in which there is no distinct terminal (R') positive deflection- and by the presence of a Q wave *prior* to the initial positve deflection (complex **H**). In each of these cases- the initial positive deflection predominates (i.e., there is a **taller *left* rabbit ear**)- which strongly favors a ventricular etiology for the anomalous complex.

Schematic complexes **C** - **D** - and **E** - in the Figure illustrate an *intermediate* morphologic pattern. Unfortunately, QRS morphology in lead V_1 or MCL_1 is of *no assistance* in differentiating between ventricular ectopy and aberrrant conduction when the QRS complex manifests one of these forms. Thus *despite* the presence of a taller *right* rabbit ear for each of these complexes- they fail to qualify as a "typical" RBBB pattern. Specifically- complex **D** lacks a distinct initial positive deflection- complex **E** begins with a Q wave (instead of an R or r wave)- and the negative deflection in complex **C** fails to descend all the way back to the baseline.

Problem: *PVCs or Aberrant ?*

Examine the tracing shown below. Is beat #13 a PVC- or an *aberrantly conducted* supraventricular impulse? How certain are you of your answer?

    <u>HINT</u>- Feel free to refer to page 325 in formulating your answer.

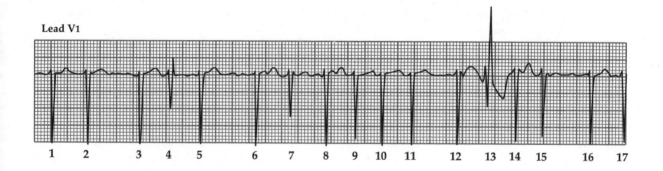

Additional Questions:

  1. What is the *underlying* rhythm in the above tracing? In the presence of this underlying rhythm- is it any more difficult to distinguish between ventricular ectopy and aberrant conduction?

  2. Can you explain the appearance of beats #4 and #7?

Answer:

As discussed in previous sections, the easiest way to interpret a complex arrhythmia in which there are several abnormalities is to determine the *underlying* rhythm first- and *then* to address the other abnormalities on the tracing. Regarding the rhythm on page 327- we therefore suggest that you initially *ignore* beats #4, 7, and 13 (since the QRS complex of these beats is clearly different from the QRS complex of all other beats on the tracing).

It can now be seen that the underlying rhythm on the preceding page is irregularly irregular- and that P waves are absent. The *underlying* rhythm is therefore **atrial fibrillation**- in this case with a fairly **rapid ventricular response** (since most R-R intervals are between 2 and 3 large boxes in duration).

The QRS complex of beats in the underlying rhythm is narrow (i.e., *not* more than *half* a large box in duration). Beat #13 is clearly widened- and very different in appearance. The question arises as to whether this beat is a PVC- or an aberrantly conducted supraventricular complex. As emphasized on page 316- a *KEY* criterion to use in making this distinction is the presence or absence of a *premature* P wave in front of the anomalous beat. Unfortunately, the presence of A Fib *precludes* using this criterion- because by definition, P waves are absent with this rhythm. Assessment of QRS morphology takes on special importance in this situation. Thus, inspection of beat #13 in the rhythm on page 327 strongly suggests **aberrant conduction**- because *all* of the characteristics of a *typical* RBBB pattern are seen for this beat. That is- beat #13 clearly manifests an rSR' pattern in this *right-sided* (V_1) lead- with a *similar* initial deflection (upright) as other supraventricular beats- an S wave that descends back down to the baseline- and an R' component that produces a taller *right* rabbit ear.

> **Note** → The reason that beats #4 and #7 on page 327 also differ in appearance- is that they are *also* aberrantly conducted. This might be suspected simply from the observation that the initial portion of these beats looks so much like the normally conducted QRS complexes. Specifically- beats #4 and #7 manifest an rSr' pattern with minimal QRS widening- that is consistent with a pattern of *incomplete* RBBB aberration.

Problem: *PVC or Aberrant ?*

Beat #4 in the tracing below seemingly manifests an rsR' pattern and *is* preceded by a P wave. *Despite these findings-* this beat is *not* aberrant. *Why not* ?

> HINT #1- Be sure to assess the regularity of the *atrial* rhythm (and determine the *timing* of the P wave preceding beat #4)!

> HINT #2- Be sure to note which monitoring *lead* is being used when assessing the significance of QRS morphology.

Lead II

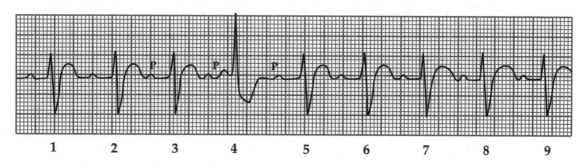

Additional Question → Is there evidence of conduction abnormality in the underlying rhythm?

Answer:

Despite the fact that beat #4 on page 329 is preceded by a P wave- and manifests a pseudo-rsR' pattern (with a taller right rabbit ear)- this beat is *not* aberrantly conducted. Instead, the *opposite* conclusion is suggested by these findings:

- Morphologic criteria for assessing the presence of a *typical* RBBB pattern (with an rsR' complex) are only valid when using a *right-sided* monitoring lead (V_1 or MCL_1). The presence of an rsR' pattern in *any other lead* is meaningless- as it is in this case because the rhythm on page 329 is recorded from lead II. Morphology of this beat #4 is *not* really suggestive of aberrant conduction, because the small initial r wave deflection is rounded and the s wave does *not* descend back down to the baseline *(see page 325).*

- The atrial (P wave) rhythm is fairly *regular* throughout the tracing. Thus, despite the fact that the anomalous complex *is* preceded by a P wave- it is *not* preceded by a *premature* P wave. Instead, the P wave preceding beat #4 occurs *on time.* The fact that the PR interval preceding this beat is so much *shorter* than the normal PR interval (which is 0.22 second in this rhythm strip) provides incontrovertible evidence that *something* else must have occurred *before* the normal atrial impulse was able to conduct. Although this "something else" could conceivably be a PJC that conducts aberrantly- this possibility is exceedingly rare. For practical purposes then- the regular atrial rate and short PR interval preceding beat #4 virtually *proves* that this widened complex is a PVC.

As emphasized on page 320- a final point in favor of a ventricular etiology for beat #4 is that there is absolutely *no reason* to expect that beat #4 should conduct with aberration- since this complex occurs so late in the cycle.

Note → Two other signs of conduction abnormality are evident on this tracing: 1) prolongation of the PR interval for the underlying rhythm (to 0.22 second- consistent with 1° AV block); and 2) prolongation of the QRS complex of sinus conducted beats (consistent with some type of bundle branch block).

Problem: *PVCs or Aberrant ?*

- When the QRS is not upright in V_1/MCL_1 -

Examine the tracing shown below. Do beats #7-9 constitute a 3-beat run of ventricular tachycardia- *or are these beats aberrantly conducted ?*

> HINT- Remember that aberrancy need *not* always manifest a pattern
> of RBBB conduction.

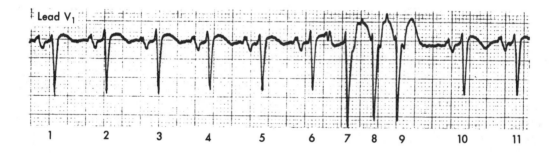

Additional Question → Other than QRS morphology- what *other* findings are present in the above tracing that might suggest aberrant conduction for beats #7-9?

> HINT- Look carefully at the T wave that immediately *precedes* the
> run of anomalous beats (i.e., the T wave of beat #6).

Answer:

It is important to emphasize that the process of differentiating between ventricular ectopy and aberrant conduction is far from perfect. Rather than providing a definitive answer in every case- our *realistic* clinical impression will much more often be expressed in terms of a *relative* probability statement (i.e., that a beat or beats is *probably* ventricular in etiology- or *probably* aberrant). So it is with this case.

We emphasized the importance of looking for a *typical* RBBB (rsR') pattern in a *right-sided* lead on pages 325-326. As helpful as the presence or absence of these morphologic features are- they can *only* be looked for when the QRS complex of the anomalous (widened) beat(s) is *upright* in lead V_1 or MCL_1. When the QRS complex of the anomalous beat(s) is predominantly *negative* in a right-sided lead (as it is for beats #7-9 on page 331)- *other* criteria must be used.

The *KEY* to this case lies with careful inspection of the T wave that *immediately* precedes the run of anomalous beats (i.e., the T wave of beat #6). Note that this T wave is definitely *notched*- whereas T waves of *all other beats* on the tracing are smooth. The presence of this T wave notching provides *telltale* evidence that a PAC must be hidden *within* this T wave- and strongly suggests that beats #7-9 must be **aberrantly conducted** supraventricular complexes.

Other fndings in support of this impression are that a "reason" *does* exist for aberrant conduction to occur here (since the PAC in the T wave of beat #6 clearly occurs at an *early* enough point in the cycle to produce aberration)- and that the QRS complex of the anomalous beats is *not* excessively widened. In general, the *wider* and more *bizarre* in appearance an anomalous beat is- the more likely it is to be *ventricular* in etiology.

> **_Beyond the Core (!!!)_** → The reason most PVCs tend to be *upright* in leads V_1 and MCL_1- is that PVCs most often originate from the *left* ventricle (and therefore depolarize in a direction oriented *toward* right-sided leads). Right ventricular PVCs are far less common- and manifest a predominantly *negative* configuration in leads V_1 and MCL_1- which must be distinguished from the pattern of *LBBB* aberration that was seen in the tracing just discussed (on page 331).

Left-Sided Lead Morphology

- *Use of Left-Sided Leads V$_6$ or MCL$_6$* -

On pages 325-326- we emphasized the diagnostic importance of using morphologic clues in a *right-sided* (V$_1$ or MCL$_1$) lead to help in differentiating between ventricular ectopy and aberrant conduction. Use of **LEFT-sided** leads (V$_6$ or MCL$_6$) may be *equally* helpful in the diagnostic process.

	Suggestive of a SUPRAVENTRICULAR Etiology/A berration	Of NO HELP in Differentiation	Suggestive of a VENTRICULAR Etiology
Left-sided monitoring leads (such as I,V5,V6 or MCL6)		 I	 J K

Question → Would you expect electrical activity associated with complex **K** (in the Figure above) to be traveling *toward* or *away* from a *left-sided* monitoring lead?

> HINT- Electrical activity that travels *toward* a monitoring lead records a *positive* QRS deflection. It records a *negative* QRS deflection when electrical activity travels *away* from the monitoring lead.

Answer:

The validity of morphologic criteria for differentiating between ventricular ectopy and aberrant conduction is supported by electrophysiologic study in which clinical correlation has been made repeatedly between QRS appearance (on an ECG)- and *definitive* identification in the laboratory. Clearly- morphologic criteria are *not* 100% reliable. However, they do provide *guidelines* that assist in our ability to predict the *relative* likelihood that an anomalous complex is *ventricular* in etiology- or *supraventricular* with aberrant conduction.

Mechanistically- the reason why morphologic criteria work is that aberrant conduction will most often manifest the pattern of *some form* of bundle branch block and/or hemiblock. As emphasized on page 322- aberrantly conducted beats most often take the form of a *typical* complete RBBB. This is because under normal circumstances, the refractory period of the right bundle branch tends to be *longer* than the refractory period of the other two major conduction fascicles. Aberrant conduction may also take the form of block in *other parts* of the conduction system (including LAHB or LPHB aberration- complete LBBB aberration- and/or *any combination* thereof). Thus, when analyzing the appearance of anomalous beats- ventricular ectopy is strongly suggested when QRS morphology is *not* consistent with *some type* of bundle branch block or hemiblock.

Full description of all nuances for the various morphologic criteria extends beyond the scope of this book. We limit discussion here to recognition of the most commonly used (and most easily remembered) criteria. These include the finding of a typical RBBB pattern in a *right-sided* lead (page 325)- and QRS appearance in a **LEFT-sided lead**. Given that the heart lies in the *left* side of the chest- one should reasonably expect *at least some* electrical activity to be directed *toward* the heart (i.e., *toward* a left-sided monitoring lead)- <u>IF</u> electrical activity is traveling *within* the ventricular conduction system (as it should be with aberrant conduction). The finding of a *totally negative* (or *almost* totally negative) QRS complex in lead V_6 or MCL_6 (i.e., complex **J** or **K** on page 333) implies that this is *not* happening- and strongly suggests a ventricular etiology.

Other patterns that *lack* a predominant negative deflection in a *left-sided* lead (such as the biphasic pattern of complex **I**)- are *not* helpful in differentiation.

Problem: *VT or not ?*

- *Using History/Statistics/Morphology/Axis* -

Examine the 12-lead ECG shown below. This tracing was obtained from a 60 year-old man with a history of prior myocardial infarction. The patient was alert and hemodynamically stable at the time this ECG was recorded. *Is this likely to be ventricular tachycardia?*

> HINT #1- Remember to use the *4 Question Approach*. Feel free to refer back to page 181 in formulating your differential diagnosis.

> HINT #2- Be sure to consider clues in the *history* given above.

> HINT #3- Be sure to also consider *morphological* clues (See page 333).

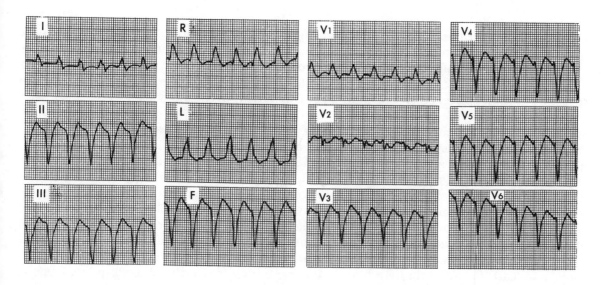

Answer:

The easiest way to interpet the rhythm on a 12-lead ECG (such as the one that appears on page 335)- is to first focus on lead II, since this is the lead that most often displays P waves the best. Doing so suggests the complete *absence* of atrial activity. Perusal of the remaining 11 leads on the tracing also fails to reveal atrial activity. The overall rhythm is rapid, regular- and the QRS complex is clearly widened. By the *4 Question Approach*- we can therefore say that there is a **regular WIDE-complex tachycardia** of **uncertain etiology**. As emphasized on page 181- there are 5 principal entities to consider:

    1. Ventricular Tachycardia (VT)
    2. *Ventricular Tachycardia*
    3. *VENTRICULAR TACHYCARDIA*
    4. SVT with aberration
    5. SVT with *pre-existing* bundle branch block (BBB)

Statistically (as suggested by the first 3 entities in the above list)- VT (*by far* !) is the most common cause of a regular *WIDE-complex* tachycardia when normal sinus P waves are nowhere to be seen. This is especially true when the **history** is that of an older adult with underlying heart disease (as is the case for the patient on page 335). One must therefore assume that the diagnosis is VT- *until proven otherwise* (and treat the patient accordingly).

Two additional clues that are easy to look for relate to the QRS axis in the frontal plane- and assessment of QRS morphology in the *KEY* leads.

Regarding **axis**- the presence of *either* a marked left or rightward axis in the frontal plane strongly supports a diagnosis of VT. Although full discussion of axis determination extends beyond the scope of this book- suffice it to say here that inspection of leads I and aVF suggests marked *left* axis deviation (given the totally *negative* deflection of the QRS complex in lead aVF).

Assessment of **QRS morphology** entails application of the principles discussed on pages 325 and 333 to the *KEY* leads used for determination of bundle branch block (i.e., *right-sided* lead V_1- and *left-sided* leads I and V_6). With regard to the rhythm on page 335- QRS morphology in lead V_1 is of little help here in differentiation (since the slurred monophasic R wave in lead V_1 lacks a definitive "rabbit ear"). However, the almost totally *negative* rS complex in lead V_6 strongly supports the diagnosis of VT.

Problem: *PVCs or Aberrant* ?

- A 2nd *Look at the Rhythm on Page 315* -

Reexamine the rhythm shown below that was used to begin this section. Apply the criteria discussed on pages 318 and 325 for diagnosing aberrant conduction. In view of the fact that this rhythm was obtained from a patient with acute myocardial infarction:

1. Would you interpret the anomalous beats as PVCs- and *therefore* consider treating the patient with lidocaine? *- or -*

2. Are these beats more likely to be *aberrantly* conducted PACs- and therefore *not* in need of antiarrhythmic treatment?

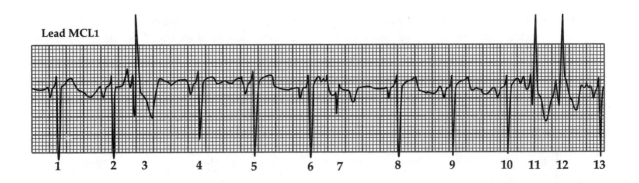

Lead MCL1

Additional Question → What degree of certainty do you place in your answer?

Answer:

The *underlying* rhythm on page 337 is **sinus**- as evidenced by the definite presence of a P wave with a constant and normal PR interval preceding each of the normal appearing beats. The negative P wave configuration seen here is common with sinus rhythm in a *right-sided* monitoring lead.

We now have ample information to declare with *virtual* **100% certainty**- that the abnormal appearing beats on this tracing (i.e., beats #3, 7, 11, and 12) are *all* **PACs** with **aberrant con-duction**:

i) Beats #3, 11, and 12 each manifest a **typical RBBB pattern** in this *right-sided* (MCL$_1$) monitoring lead. Specifically- QRS mophology is consistent with pat-terns A and B on page 325 (in that an rsR'/rSR' complex is seen- with a taller *right* rabbit ear- in which the S wave descends *below* the baseline).

ii) A **similar *initial* deflection** (in direction and slope) is seen for anomalous beats (in the form of an *upward* r wave)- as for normally conducted beats.

iii) Beats #3 and #11 are each preceded by a **premature P wave** (seen here as extra peaking in the T wave of beat #2- and *notching* in the T wave of beat #10).

iv) A **"reason"** exists for aberrant conduction. That is- anomalous beats *all* occur at an early enough point in the cardiac cycle to reasonably expect aberrant conduction.

> **Beyond the Core** → Beat #7 in the tracing on page 337 is *also* aberrantly conducted. Although different in appearance from other aberrantly conducted beats (it lacks a tall R' component)- it never-theless manifests an rSr' configuration with a similar *initial* deflection (in the form of a small, but definitely positive r wave deflection)- and is preceded by a *premature* P wave (that *notches* the T wave of beat #6). The reason beat #7 is *not* quite as wide as the other anomalous beats (that conduct with a pattern of *complete* RBBB aberration)- and the reason that beat #7 lacks a tall R' component- is that **beat #7** is con-ducted with a pattern of **incomplete RBBB aberration**.

Fusion Beats

Examine the tracing shown below. Are the anomalous beats PVCs- or aberrantly conducted? Why do you suppose that beat #8 looks so different from the other anomalous beats on this tracing?

> HINT- Is the PR interval preceding beat #8 *long enough* to allow time for conduction- or is this PR interval *shorter* than other PR intervals on the tracing?

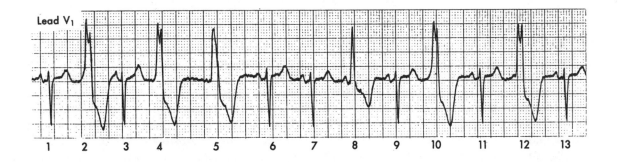

Additional Question → Is QRS morphology for anomalous beats #2, 4, 5, 10, and 12 suggestive of ventricular ectopy- or aberrant conduction?

> HINT- Feel free to refer to the Table on page 325 in formulating your answer.

Answer:

The tracing that appears on the page 339 is *not* an easy one to interpret. The *KEY* to interpretation lies with assessing the various components of the rhythm- *one at a time*.

We suggest you begin by trying to determine the *underlying* rhythm. This can most easily be done by looking to see if two *"normal"* appearing beats ever occur in a row. *They do*- for beats #6 and 7. Careful inspection of these two beats reveals that the QRS complex is narrow- and that a P wave precedes each beat with a constant and normal PR interval. With these two beats as a model for comparison- it can now be seen that there are other "normal" appearing beats on the tracing (i.e., beats #1, 3, 9, 11, and 13). Thus- *despite* the fact that many beats in the tracing are widened, bizarre in morphology, and *not* associated with P waves- the *underlying* rhythm is **sinus**.

We suggest you *defer* interpretation of beat #8 until last. Instead- look next at the most widened beats on the tracing (i.e., beats #2, 4, 5, 10, and 12). Each of these beats is a **PVC**. We say this with virtual ***100% certainty***- based on bizarre QRS morphology (with if anything, a taller *left* rabbit ear- consistent with patterns F and G on page 325)- no preceding premature P wave- and no "reason" for aberrant conduction (given the relatively *late* occurrence of each of these beats in the cardiac cycle). In fact, beat #5 occurs so late- that it would be better classified as a ventricular *escape* beat rather than a "premature" ventricular contraction.

We are left with interpretation of **beat #8**. The reason this complex looks different than the other ventricular beats on this tracing is that it represents a ***fusion* beat**- resulting from *partial* conduction of its preceding P wave through the ventricles until (somewhere in its path) it meets the wave of depolarization emanating from an almost simultaneously occurring PVC. Fusion beats therefore manifest characteristics of *both* the *supraventricular* impulse (i.e., sinus beat)- and the *ventricular* beat (i.e., the PVC). Simply stated- if beats #7 and #10 were to "have children"- *one of the offspring might look like beat #8.*

> **KEY** → The clinical significance of recognizing *fusion* beats on a tracing- is that this finding *proves* a ventricular etiology for the widened beats.

AV Dissociation

Examine the tracing shown below. Note that the atrial (P wave) rhythm remains *regular* throughout the tracing (*arrows* indicating a regular P-P interval of just over 3 large boxes in duration). *Can you explain what is happening*?

HINT- Remember the causes of a *WIDE-complex* tachycardia.

Lead II

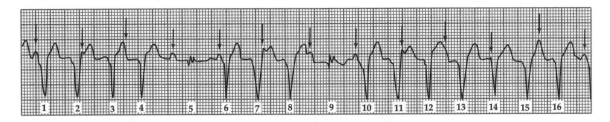

Additional Question → Are *any* P waves shown above being conducted to the ventricles?

Answer:

The *underlying* mechanism for the rhythm shown on page 341 is *not* readily apparent from initial inspection of the tracing. Nevertheless, application of the *4 Question Approach* greatly facilitates interpretation.

The basic rhythm is composed of QS complexes that are *widened* and *regular* at a rate of 135 beats/minute. Two "different-looking" complexes (beats #5 and 9) *interrupt* this underlying rhythm. The first of these complexes (i.e., beat #5) is preceded by a P wave that appears to be conducting- albeit with 1° AV block. Scanning the rest of the tracing for signs of atrial activity reveals *peaking* and *notching* at various points in the cardiac cycle. *Setting one's calipers* to the interval defined by *two* of these points (i.e., to the interval defined by the P wave preceding beat #5- and the positive deflection *just before* beat #6)- allows atrial activity to be *"marched out"* across the tracing (*arrows*). Thus- an underlying *regular* atrial rhythm is present! Because this atrial activity is for the most part *unrelated* to the QRS complex- **AV dissociation** is present- in which the negative complexes (with a QS configuration) represent runs of **ventricular tachycardia** that are *interrupted* by **sinus capture beats** (beats #5 and #9). The q waves of these sinus-conducted beats and the 1° AV block are each manifestations of this patient's acute *inferior* myocardial infarction.

> **KEY →** Although clearly a <u>difficult</u> tracing to interpret- the point to emphasize is the diagnostic value of looking for a "break" in the rhythm. Subtle atrial activity will often be seen best *during* such relative pauses in the rhythm (such as the one that occurs here between beats #4-6).
>
> Clinically- the importance of recognizing AV dissociation (and/or sinus capture beats) is that these findings provide strong evidence in favor of a *ventricular* etiology for a tachyarrhythmia. Unfortunately, these findings are *only* seen in a minority of cases of VT.

Beyond the Core! → Despite the fact that the PR interval preceding beat #9 is *longer* than the PR interval preceding beat #5- *both* beats are probably being conducted. The reason the PR interval preceding beat #9 is longer is probably due to the *earlier* occurrence of this P wave in the cardiac cycle (which impairs conduction through the AV node- and prolongs the PR interval of the subsequent beat).

<u>Review:</u> *PVCs or Aberrant ?*

The underlying rhythm in the tracing shown below is atrial fibrillation. Every other beat occurs early and is widened. *Is every other beat a PVC- or aberrantly conducted ?*

> <u>HINT</u>- Note that the **coupling interval** (i.e., the interval *between* normal appearing complexes and the subsequent widened beat) is constant. *Would you expect this with atrial fibrillation ?*

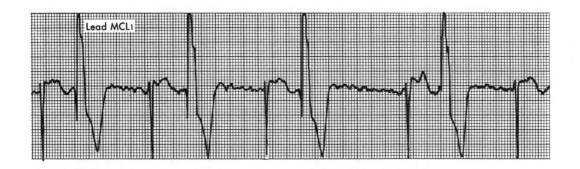

<u>Additional Question</u> → Is QRS morphology of the anomalous beats more suggestive of ventricular ectopy- or aberrant conduction?

> <u>HINT</u>- Feel free to refer to the Table on page 325 in formulating your answer.

Answer:

As noted at the top of page 343- the *underlying* rhythm in the tracing shown is **atrial fib-rillation** (evidenced by the erratic baseline and lack of definite P waves). A wide and bizarre looking QRS complex occurs every other beat. The question arises as to whether these anomalous complexes are PVCs- or aberrantly conducted supraventricular impulses.

Because the underlying rhythm is A Fib, the diagnostic value of looking for a premature P wave is lost. This is because by definition, P waves are absent with this rhythm. Nevertheless- *other* factors strongly favor a *ventricular* etiology for the beats in question. These include:

    i) The presence of *fixed* coupling in association with A Fib.
    ii) QRS morphology in this *right-sided* (MCL_1) monitoring lead
    iii) Marked QRS widening of the beats in question.

If the anomalous complexes were supraventricular impulses that conducted with aberration- one would certainly expect them to occur with the same *irregular irregularity* as the underlying rhythm. This is in contrast to what most often happens with PVCs. In particular, PVCs that manifest a similar ECG appearance most probably arise from the same ectopic focus. Because the most common mechanism of ventricular ectopy is **reentry** (through a well-defined circuit of myocardial cells)- uniform PVCs will tend to have a constant coupling interval. Thus, in the presence of A Fib- the finding of anomalous beats with a *fixed* coupling interval (as seen here) is strongly suggestive of ventricular ectopy.

QRS morphology is also consistant with a ventricular etiology. Specifically- the first three anomalous beats manifest a QR-"slur" configuration with taller *left* rabbit ear (that most closely resembles pattern H on page 325). In addition, the initial deflection of these first three anomalous beats is *oppositely* directed (i.e., negative) to the small positive r wave of the normally conducted beats. The last anomalous complex is equally bizarre with an rR-"slur" configuration (that more closely resembles patterns F or G on page 325). Finally- the *marked* degree of QRS widening for anomalous complexes (that we estimate to be *at least* 0.15 second) is also consistent with ventricular ectopy- since aberrantly conducted complexes tend to manifest lesser degrees of QRS widening.

<u>Review:</u> *PVCs or Aberrant ?*

The tracing below is a ***bigeminal* rhythm** in which every other beat is widened and markedly different in morphology. *Are the anomalous beats PVCs- or aberrantly conducted?*

> <u>HINT</u>- Always assume that a beat is "guilty" (i.e., a PVC)- until *proven* "innocent" (i.e., *aberrantly* conducted).

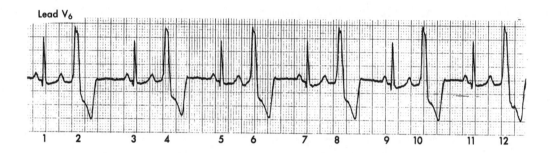

<u>Additional Question</u> → Is there any way to determine what a "normal" T wave looks like with a *bigeminal* rhythm? That is- do two *normal* (i.e., sinus-conducted) beats ever occur in a row?

Answer:

The *underlying* rhythm on page 345 is **sinus**- as evidenced by the presence of normal appearing P waves with a constant PR interval in front of each of the odd numbered beats. Every other beat is markedly widened and very different in appearance. In addition, the initial deflection of anomalous beats is not only oppositely directed, but also very different (more gradual) in slope- further supporting our already strong impression that these beats must be **PVCs**.

Unfortunately, one problem inherent with trying to interpret a *bigeminal* rhythm is that because every other beat is different- it may be quite difficult (if not impossible) to determine if premature P waves might be buried within preceding T waves. That is- because we *never* see two normal sinus-conducted beats occur in a row, there is no way to know what a "normal" T wave should look like. There is therefore no way to tell for sure if the T wave preceding each anomalous complex is being deformed by a PAC. This problem is solved in this case by the rhythm shown below- obtained a short while later from the same patient.

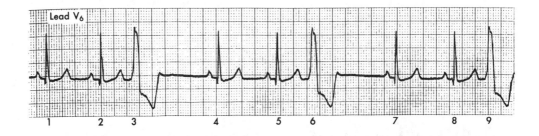

Note that there is now a **trigeminal rhythm**- in which every *third* beat is anomalous. Consecutive normal (i.e., sinus-conducted) beats now occur. Focusing attention on the "normal" T waves that are seen in this tracing (i.e., the T waves of beats #1, 4, and 7)- and comparing these normal T waves to the T waves that precede the anomalous beats (i.e., the T waves of beats #2, 5, and 8)- we can now be more comfortable concluding that premature P waves are *not* subtly hiding within preceding T waves. The anomalous beats *must* therefore be **PVCs**- and we interpret these rhythms as **ventricular *bigeminy* and *trigeminy*.**

<u>Review:</u> *PVCs or Aberrant* ?

Examine the tracing shown below, obtained from a patient with acute myocardial infarction. Are the three anomalous beats likely to be PVCs- *or PACs that are aberrantly conducted* ?

> <u>HINT #1</u>- Remember that *not* all of the rules work all of the time.

> <u>HINT #2</u>- Be sure to look *carefully* at the T wave preceding each anomalous beat. Is this T wave the *same* as the T wave of the *other* sinus conducted beats?

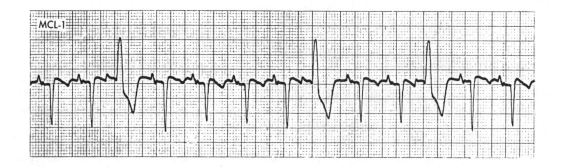

<u>KEY Clinical Question</u> → Given the setting of acute myocardial infarction- should *new-onset* anomalous beats of the nature shown above be treated with lidocaine?

Answer:

The *underlying* rhythm on page 347 is **sinus tachycardia** at a rate of 105 beats/minute. Unfortunately, morphologic assessment of the anomalous beats in this tracing (as illustrated on page 325) is *not* of much assistance in diagnosis. This is because an initial r wave is absent. Anomalous beats on this tracing therefore manifest an *intermediate* morphologic pattern (with a qR configuration that most closely resembles complex **E** on page 325). The reason the initial positive deflection (r wave) is missing may be as a result of the acute infarction. However, because the normally conducted sinus beats *also* lack an initial r wave- a *typical* RBBB pattern might not occur for the anomalous beats even if aberration was present. Therefore- *no conclusions* can be drawn regarding etiology of these anomalous beats based on morphologic assessment.

On the other hand- *premature* atrial activity *does* clearly precede each anomalous complex. Even in the absence of suggestive morphologic features, the finding of *definite* **PACs** that precede each anomalous beat provides very strong evidence in favor of **aberrant conduction**.

The *KEY* to recognizing the presence of *premature* atrial activity is to direct one's attention first at determining the appearance of a "normal" T wave. Then compare this normal T wave appearance- with the appearance of those T waves that *immediately* precede each anomalous beat. Doing so reveals the *"telltale"* notching of a PAC that is buried *within* (and *deforms*) the T wave preceding each anomalous beat. The fact that this finding is so consistent (i.e., the *only* T waves on this tracing that are notched are the ones that immediately precede each anomalous beat)- supports our contention that this finding is *real* (and is *not* the result of artifact).

KEY → Not all of the rules for aberrant conduction are present all of the time. The tracing on the front of this card is an excellent example of how aberrant conduction can sometimes be diagnosed with relative certainty- *despite* the absence of suggestive morphologic features. As a result of this diagnosis, the patient should *not* be treated with lidocaine (since PACs do *not* place the patient at increased risk). In contrast- *new-onset* ventricular ectopy in the setting of acute ischemic heart disease *may* merit treatment.

Review: *VT or not* **?**

The tracing below shows a tachyarrhythmia with QRS widening. *Is this ventricular tachycardia* ?

> HINT- Be sure to consider the *regularity* of the rhythm (and/or the *lack* thereof) in formulating your answer.

Lead II

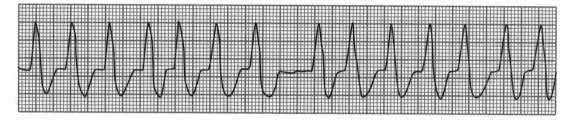

Additional Question → How might a *supraventricular* tachycardia produce QRS widening?

> HINT- You have *already* seen the above rhythm (and answered this question) on pages 187-188.

Answer:

The rhythm that appears on page 349 is a *WIDE-complex* tachycardia (WCT). As repeatedly emphasized throughout this book- it is essential to *always* strongly consider the possibility of ventricular tachycardia (VT)- *whenever* you encounter a WCT of *uncertain* etiology. However, *despite* this precaution- the rhythm on page 349 is *unlikely* to be VT.

Our reason for suspecting that VT is *not* present in this case is based on assessment of the regularity of this rhythm- or more precisely, the *lack* thereof. VT is usually a regular (or at least *almost* regular) rhythm. This is in contrast to what is seen for the tracing on the preceding page- in which R-R intervals vary *continually* from beat to beat. In conjunction with the complete absence of atrial activity- it becomes much more likely that the rhythm on page 349 represents **atrial fibrillation** rather than VT. QRS widening would then be explained by presuming the presence of *pre-existing* bundle branch block. (Access to a prior 12-lead ECG is therefore *invaluable* for confirming that preexisting bundle branch block does or does not exist.)

> **Note** → Assessment of QRS morphology is of no assistance for interpreting the rhythm on page 349- because this tracing is recorded from lead II. Thus, despite our strong suspicion that this rhythm represents A Fib (because of its irregular irregularity)- it is impossible to make this diagnosis with certainty on the basis of this single tracing alone.

Review: *VT or not* ?

Examine the 12-lead ECG shown below. This tracing was obtained from an older adult with a long prior history of ischemic heart disease. The patient was alert and hemodynamically stable at the time this ECG was recorded. *Is this likely to be ventricular tachycardia?*

> HINT- Feel free to refer to our discussion on pages 335-336 in formulating your answer.

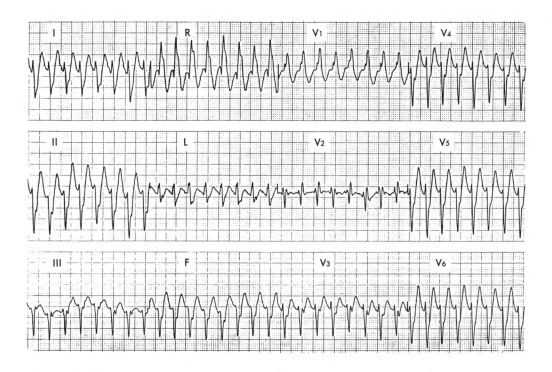

Answer:

The tracing and clinical scenario described on page 351 closely resemble the situation presented earlier on page 335. The clinical approach to evaluation and management should be the
same.

The easiest way to begin interpretation is to focus attention first on lead II (since this is the
lead that most often displays P waves the best). Doing so fails to reveal evidence of atrial activity. Scanning each of the remaining 11 leads on the tracing for atrial activity similarly fails to
reveal any sign of P waves. The overall rhythm on this ECG is rapid, regular- and the QRS complex is clearly widened. We therefore define this rhythm as a **regular *WIDE-complex* tachycardia (WCT)** of ***uncertain etiology***. Several points should be emphasized:

i) VT *must* be assumed as the etiology of the rhythm- until *proven* otherwise.

ii) Clinically- the patient's *hemodynamic status* is the most important factor for
determining how to proceed. This is because if the patient shows any sign of
hemodynamic compromise in association with the rhythm (i.e., hypotension,
chest pain, shortness of breath, and/or mental confusion)- it will *no longer*
matter what the rhythm really is. Synchronized cardioversion now becomes
immediately indicated- *regardless* of whether the rhythm turns out to be VT
(or SVT with aberrant conduction).

iii) Clinical parameters (i.e., the patient's age and long prior history of ischemic
heart disease)- are both consistent with a *ventricular* etiology in this case.

iv) Assessment of other factors (i.e., mean QRS axis and morphologic features)-
provide further support in favor of VT. Specifically- the presence of *marked*
axis deviation (leftward, rightward- and/or *indeterminate*)- strongly suggests
a ventricular etiology. The presence of deeply negative QRS complexes in *both*
leads I and aVF defines the axis here as indeterminate.

Morphologically- the r-slur-R' configuration in lead V_1 (consistent with
patterns C and D on page 325)- is *not* helpful diagnostically. However, the
predominantly *negative* QRS deflection in lead V_6 (that most closely resembles pattern **J** on page 333)- strongly suggests VT.

v) VT is (*by far!*) the most common cause of a WCT of *uncertain* etiology.

Review: *VT or not ?*

Examine the 12-lead ECG shown below. This tracing was obtained from an older adult with a long prior history of congestive heart failure. The patient was in pulmonary edema at the time this ECG was recorded. *Is this likely to be ventricular tachycardia* ?

> HINT- Be sure to assess the *regularity* of this rhythm (and/or the lack thereof) in *all* 12 leads- *before* formulating your answer.

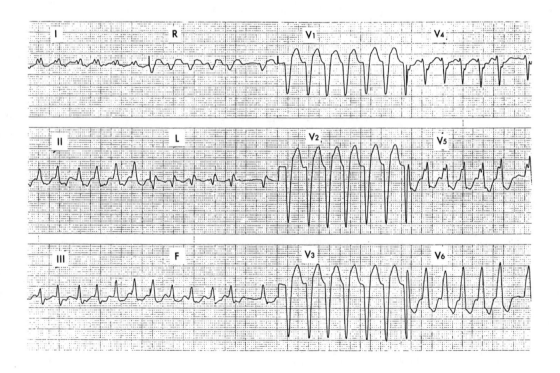

Answer:

Once again- the rhythm that appears on page 353 is a *WIDE-complex* tachycardia. The frontal plane axis is normal. QRS morphology is *not* helpful diagnostically in this example- as it could be consistent with *either* a supraventricular or ventricular etiology. Although there are fine undulations in the baseline- no definite atrial activity is seen. However, in contrast to the ECG we reviewed on page 351- the underlying rhythm in this tracing is *not* regular. Instead, it is *irregularly irregular*- especially in simultaneously recorded leads aVR, aVL, and aVF. The presence of an irregularly irregular rhythm *without* definite atrial activity suggests that the rhythm is **atrial fibrillation**- in this case with a moderately rapid ventricular response. QRS widening would then be explained on the basis of *preexisting* LBBB.

Several points should be emphasized regarding interpretation of this ECG:

i) Although we strongly suspect that the rhythm is A Fib (with QRS widening from *preexisting* bundle branch block)- it is difficult to be certain of this diagnosis from inspection of *only* this tracing. Locating a previous ECG on this patient to verify the presence of preexisting bundle branch block would be invaluable for confirming the diagnosis.

ii) Recognition of the irregularity of A Fib may be difficult when the ventricular response to this rhythm is rapid (as it is in this case). Careful measurement of successive R-R intervals (ideally with *calipers*) would greatly facilitate diagnosis.

iii) Assessment of QRS morphology is *not* really helpful in this case. This is because the diagnostic criteria for QRS morphology that we described on page 325 can *not* be applied when the QRS complex is *not* predominantly upright in lead V_1. As noted on pages 333-334- the upright QRS complex seen here in lead V_6 on page 353 is consistent with *either* a supraventricular or ventricular etiology.

A Brief Look
at Pediatric Arrhythmias

- Pediatric Cardiopulmonary Arrest -

Although the terminology used to define pediatric and adult arrhythmias is similar- the spectrum of rhythm disorders encountered and priorities for evaluation and management differ significantly. **Children are *not* just little adults!**

The intricacies of interpreting pediatric arrhythmias extend well beyond the scope of this book. Nevertheless, it may still be helpful to emphasize certain *KEY* points regarding pediatric arrhythmias. We begin by reflecting on the rhythms encountered with pediatric resuscitation.

Question ➔ What are the most common arrhythmias associated with pediatric cardiopulmonary arrest? How does this differ from cardiopulmonary arrest in adults?

> HINT- What is the most common *underlying* cause of cardiopulmonary arrest in infants and children?

Answer:

By far- the most common cause of pediatric cardiopulmonary arrest is *inadequate oxygenation* with resultant *hypoxemia.* In response to this hypoxemia- the pediatric heart tends to *slow* its rate. Marked bradycardia is often seen. Common *preterminal* rhythms in infants and children therefore include profound sinus bradycardia and/or arrhythmia, sinus arrest with slow junctional or idioventricular escape, and other bradycardia with AV block. Asystole is the most common *terminal* event. It should be noted that this is in direct contrast to what occurs with cardiopulmonary arrest in adults- for whom ventricular tachyarrhythmias (especially VT and V Fib) are most commonly seen. VT and V Fib are only *rarely* seen in pediatric cardiopulmonary arrest.

With regard to the management of cardiopulmonary arrest in infants and children, the following points should be emphasized:

i) Establishing a patent airway that allows adequate ventilation and oxygenation (enhanced by supplemental oxygen) is the *KEY* to success- and will often be all that is needed. This is why **Oxygen** is the *most* important drug (*by far!*) in pediatric resuscitation.

ii) In addition to hypoxemia- other factors that are likely to contribute to pediatric cardiopulmonary arrest/arrhythmogenesis include acidosis, hypotension, electrolyte disturbance, hypoglycemia, hypothermia, and/or the presence of an underlying illness (i.e., sepsis, pneumonia, dehydration, etc.). Correction of underlying disorders is a second important *KEY* for successful resuscitation.

iii) In those cases when pharmacologic therapy *is* needed in pediatric resuscitation- the *most* important agent to consider is **Epinephrine**. Atropine may be useful at times- but is now considered a *second-line* agent for treatment of pediatric bradyarrhythmias.

iv) Defibrillation is only *rarely* needed in pediatric cardiopulmonary arrest. This is because as noted above- *bradycardia* is by far the most common response of the pediatric heart to cardiopulmonary arrest.

Pediatric Norms

- *Norms for Heart Rate/Intervals* -

The rhythm strip shown below was obtained from a 6 month old infant. It shows **sinus rhythm**- but at a heart rate of 140 beats/minute. The PR interval is 0.11 second- and the QRS interval is 0.05 second. *Are these parameters (for heart rate and intervals) normal for a pediatric patient ?*

Lead II

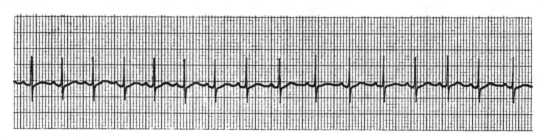

Additional Question → How would you assess the clinical significance of the above rhythm?

Answer:

Pediatric norms for heart rate and interval (PR and QRS) duration differ markedly from those of adults. As a result, the tracing that appears on page 357 (if obtained from a healthy infant)- would be completely normal!

Pediatric Norms- are shown in the Table below:

Age	Heart Rate (beats/minute)	PR Interval (second)	QRS Duration (second)
Newborn- 1 yr	90-180	0.07-0.16	0.03-0.08
1-3 yrs old	70-150	0.08-0.16	0.04-0.08
4-10 yrs old	60-130	0.09-0.17	0.04-0.09
> 10 yrs old	60-110	0.09-0.20	0.04-0.09

From this Table- it can be seen that heart rates of *up to* 180 beats/minute are still *normal* for children during the first year of life. During this time, *mean* heart rate is between 120-140 beats/minute. Heart rates below 90 beats/minute constitute sinus *bradycardia* (although it would *not* be uncommon or abnormal for the heart rate of an otherwise healthy infant to drop below 80 beats/minute during sleep). Clearly- the *most* important factor (*by far!*) for determining the clinical significance of any pediatric arrhythmia- is the *clinical setting* in which it occurs. Sinus tachycardia at a rate of 200 beats/minute (or more)- may be entirely normal in an otherwise healthy young child who is vigorously crying. In contrast- a sinus rate of 70 beats/minute would be inappropriately slow for an acutely ill child of the same age- and may reflect inadequate oxygenation.

> **Practice** → Verify in the above Table that for a **6-month old infant**- the parameters noted for the rhythm on page 357 (i.e., a heart rate of 140 beats/minute; PR interval = 0.11 second; QRS interval = 0.05 second)- are all *normal* !
>
> Note also from the Table above that for a **3-year old child**- a PR interval of 0.18 second is *long* (= 1° AV block!)- and a QRS interval of 0.09 second is *wide* !

Subsidiary Pacemakers

- Pediatric Norms for Escape Rhythms -

The sinoatrial (SA) node is the principal pacemaker of the heart. Under normal circumstances, it suppresses all other cardiac tissue with its inherent automaticity. In an awake child with normal sinus rhythm- the SA node fires at a rate of between 60-180 beats/minute (depending on the age and activity of the child- as shown in the Table on page 358).

Question → What would you expect to happen if for any reason the principal pacemaker (i.e., SA node) *fails* to fire?

- How might the situation differ for a child compared to an adult?

Answer:

If for any reason the principal pacemaker of the heart (the SA node) either *slows* markedly or *fails* to fire at all- another (*subsidiary*) pacemaker will be charged with taking over. The resulting rhythm is known as an **escape rhythm**.

The Table below shows the usual escape rates of **subsidiary pacemakers** in the atria, AV node, and ventricles for children and adults.

Site of Escape Focus	Up to 3 Years Old (beats/minute)	Over 3 Years Old & Adults (beats/minute)
Atria	80-100	50-60
AV node	50-80	40-60
Ventricles	40-50	20-40

According to this Table- were the sinus rate to slow down in a child *less* than 3 years of age- a subsidiary pacemaker in the atria might take over at a rate of between 80 to 100 beats/minute. If this did not occur, one would then expect an escape rhythm to arise from the site that was *"next in line"* in the pacemaking hierarchy- which is the AV node. For a child under 3- the usual rate of a subsidiary pacemaker from this site is between 50 to 80 beats/minute. The lowest escape focus- a site in the ventricles- is left as a final safeguard in the event no escape rhythm is forthcoming from either the atria or AV node. The rate of an idioventricular escape rhythm in a child under 3 is usually between 40 to 50 beats/minute. As can be seen from the Table- *the rate of subsidiary pacemakers for children after about 3 years of age is similar to that for adults.*

> **Note** → Escape rhythms are extremely common in otherwise healthy children- and usually do *not* represent a disease state. This is particularly true for escape rhythms that occur during sleep (when variations in vagal tone frequently result in sinus slowing and transient AV nodal escape).

Problem: *What is the rhythm ?*

The tracing shown below developed suddenly in a previously healthy 4-year old child. What entities should be considered in your differential diagnosis?

> HINT- Feel free to refer back to page 125- remembering that diagnostic considerations will be somewhat *different* for children.

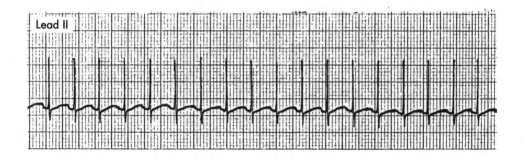

Additional Question → Does the heart rate in the above example exceed 200 beats/minute?

> HINT- You may want to apply the *Every-OTHER-Beat Method* (discussed on pages 55-58) in formulating your answer.

Answer:

The rhythm that appears on page 361 is rapid and regular. By the *Every-OTHER-Beat Method-* we estimate the heart rate to be *just under* 200 beats/minute (since the R-R interval of every *other* beat is *just over* 3 large boxes in duration). The QRS complex in this rhythm is definitely *narrow-* and no sign of atrial activity is seen. Thus, the rhythm represents a regular *narrow-complex* (i.e., *supraventricular*) tachycardia. Diagnostic considerations in the pediatric age group for a **Regular SVT** include:

> 1. Sinus tachycardia
> 2. Atrial flutter
> 3. PSVT
> 4. Ectopic atrial tachycardia (EAT)

Note that the fourth entity listed above (EAT) was *not* included among the most common causes of a regular SVT in adults (that we listed on page 125)- as this rhythm is only rarely seen outside the pediatric age group.

Clinical correlation is needed to determine the cause of the tachycardia in this case. Clearly, the rate of ≈195 beats/minute that is seen here is more rapid than what one usually expects for sinus tachycardia- although rates of up to 220 beats/minute have been recorded in children! Nevertheless, the absence of atrial activity- and the fact that this child was perfectly well prior to the sudden onset of this arrhythmia both argue against a diagnosis of sinus tachycardia. *Children with rapid sinus tachycardia are almost always ill from some other cause* !

Atrial flutter is an uncommon rhythm in children. This is fortunate from a diagnostic standpoint because the rate parameters characteristic of atrial flutter in adults do *not* hold true in children (for whom the flutter rate often exceeds 300/minute- and the ventricular response is often irregular).

Distinction between EAT and PSVT is often difficult from a single rhythm strip. The former diagnosis is far less common, and usually more gradual in onset. Thus, relative frequency statistics *and* the history in this case (i.e., that the child was previously well- and that the arrhythmia developed abruptly)- are both in favor of **PSVT** as the diagnosis.

Problem: *What is the rhythm ?*

Examine the tracing shown below, obtained from a 2-year old child. Is the sixth beat *wide enough* to be a PVC?

> <u>HINT</u>- Feel free to refer back to the Table on page 358 in formulating your
> answer.

Lead II

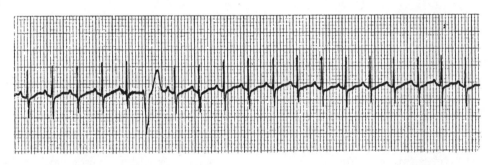

<u>Additional Question</u> → Why do you suppose PVCs in children are
not as wide as PVCs in adults?

Answer:

The *underlying* rhythm that appears on page 363 is **sinus tachycardia** at a rate of about 200 beats/minute. The sixth complex differs markedly from all other beats on the tracing- and is *not* preceded by a P wave. Clearly this beat is a **PVC**. Yet it measures *at most* no more than 0.09 second in duration.

As noted in the Table on page 358- QRS interval duration is normally between 0.04-0.08 second for a 2-year old child. Thus, the sixth complex on page 363 *is* wide- considering the age of this patient. The reason why PVCs tend to be *narrower* in children than in adults is simply a result of the fact that the ectopic impulse requires less time to travel through the smaller pediatric heart.

Note → From the above example, one can easily imagine how ventricular tachycardia in a child might be mistaken by an adult-oriented emergency care provider as a supraventricular tachycardia. *Wide* is a relative term. It is important to remember that 0.09-0.10 second represents definite QRS widening in children. At the extreme- a case of VT has been reported in a newborn infant in which the QRS complex of the tachyarrhythmia was *only* 0.05 second !!!!

Practically speaking- the diagnostic dilemmas described above will not be encountered often by most emergency care providers- since ventricular tachyarrhythmias are relatively uncommon in pediatric patients.

Problem: *What is the rhythm ?*

Examine the tracing shown below. Is the presence of *group beating* indicative of Mobitz I (Wenckebach) 2° AV block?

> HINT #1- The tracing was obtained from a completely healthy and playful young child.

> HINT #2- We have *already* seen this rhythm (on page 289).

Lead II

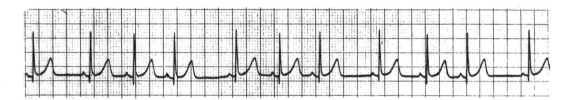

Answer:

Despite the presence of *group beating* in the rhythm that appears on page 365- this is *not* a manifestation of AV Wenckebach. None of the other *KEY* "footprints" of Wenckebach (that we discussed on page 267-268) are seen. That is- the atrial rate is *not* regular- the PR interval does *not* prolong- and the duration of the pause is *not* less than twice the shortest R-R interval.

Instead, the mechanism of the rhythm on page 365 is *sinus*- as evidenced by the fact that each QRS complex is preceded by a normal appearing (upright) P wave in this lead II recording with a fixed (and normal) PR interval. The QRS complex is of normal duration. Thus, the irregularity in this rhythm is a result of **sinus arrhythmia**- an extremely common *normal* finding in healthy children and young adults (in whom heart rate *often* varies in cyclical fashion with the pattern of respiration).

INDEX

M

Magnesium sulfate, 314
MAT; *see* Multifocal atrial tachycardia
MCL₁, QRS morphology in, 325-326
Mechanical activity in arrhythmia interpretation, 17-18, 23-24
Mobitz type I, 236, 261-262, 263-264, 266, 267-268, 279-280, 286
    vs. Mobitz type II, 277-278, 279-280, 281-282
    pediatric, 365-366
Mobitz type II, 236, 261-262, 275-276, 279-280
Moderate ventricular response, atrial fibrillation with, 105-106
Multifocal atrial tachycardia (MAT), 110, 130, 308
Multiform PVCs, 169-170

N

Narrow QRS rhythms, 101-102
Non-sustained ventricular tachycardia, 177-178, 179-180
Normal conduction, pathway of, in arrhythmia interpretation, 13-14
Normal sinus rhythm (NSR), 14, 70, 74, 84, 89-90, 144, 156, 158, 160, 193-194, 242, 301-302

O

1:1 AV conduction, 84, 176
Oxygenation, inadequate, with hypoxemia, pediatric, 356

P

P wave, 17-18, 64, 70, 83-84, 91-92, 94, 96, 98, 99-100, 104, 105-106, 109-110, 122, 126, 140, 142, 180, 184, 188, 190, 194, 204, 208, 210, 240, 242, 244, 252, 260, 266, 272, 276, 280, 284, 286, 288, 290, 292, 294, 318, 330, 338
    in 4 question approach, 62, 73-78
    biphasic, 164
    relationship between QRS complex and, in 4 question approach, 62, 83-86, 240, 242, 244, 252, 260, 272, 276, 280, 286, 288, 290, 294
P wave polarity, 75-76, 143-144, 145
Pacemakers, subsidiary, pediatric norms for escape rhythms and, 359-360
PACs; *see* Premature atrial contractions
Palpitations, 132
Paper, grid, in arrhythmia interpretation, 37-46
Paroxysmal atrial tachycardia (PAT), 128, 130
Paroxysmal junctional tachycardia (PJT), 128, 130
Paroxysmal supraventricular tachycardia (PSVT), 10, 101-102, 125-126, 127-128, 130
    clinical significance of, 131-132
    effect of carotid sinus massage on, 138
    pediatric, 362
PAT; *see* Paroxysmal atrial tachycardia
Pathway of normal conduction in arrhythmia interpretation, 13-14
Patient as component of clinical arrhythmia interpretation, 5-6
Patterns of regularity of rhythm, 65-66
PEA; *see* Pulseless electrical activity
Pediatric arrhythmias, 355-356
Pediatric cardiopulmonary arrest, 355-356
Pediatric norms, 357-358, 359-360
Pediatric rhythms, 150, 355-366
    cardiopulmonary arrest and, 355-356
    pediatric arrhythmias and, 355-356
    pediatric norms and, 357-358
    subsidiary pacemakers and, 359-360
Phenothiazine, 314
PJCs; *see* Premature junctional contractions
PJT; *see* Paroxysmal junctional tachycardia
Polarity, P wave, 75-76, 143-144, 145
P-P interval, 64, 86
PR interval, 19-20, 22, 84, 100, 122, 266, 267-268, 271-272, 287-288
Premature atrial contractions (PACs), 16, 68, 150, 153 154, 156, 159-160, 198, 274, 315-316, 324, 338, 348
    with aberration, 159-160
    blocked, 159-160, 198, 288, 324
    clinical significance of, 155-156
    diagnostic features of, 155-156
    vs. PVCs, 163-166
Premature beats, 68, 87-88, 151-190
    aberrant PACs and, 159-160
    bigeminy and, 171-172
    blocked PACs and, 159-160
    early and late beats and, 151-152
    multiform PVCs and, 169-170
    PACs and, 155-156, 163-166
    PJCs and, 157-158
    PVCs and, 161-162, 163-166
    repetitive forms of PVCs and, 167-168
    trigeminy and, 171-172
    types of, 153-154
    ventricular tachycardia and, 177-180, 185-186
    wide complex tachycardia and, 181-182

U

U wave, 17-18
Unclaimed terms, degree of AV block and, 240
Usurpation, 148, 202, 254, 292

V

V fib; *see* Ventricular fibrillation
Vagal maneuvers, 132, 134, 135-138, 139, 150
    in arrhythmia interpretation, 9-10
    carotid sinus massage and; *see* Carotid sinus
        massage
    effect of, on tachyarrhythmias, 137-138
Valsalva, 10
Variable ventricular response, 176
Ventricles
    diastolic filling of, 107-108
    escape beats arising from, 192
    escape rhythms and, 360
Ventricular arrhythmias, 80
    carotid sinus massage and, 136
    sustained, 87-88
Ventricular bigeminy, 171-172, 345-346
Ventricular contractions, premature; *see* Premature
       ventricular contractions
Ventricular couplets, 167-168, 198
Ventricular fibrillation (V fib), 24, 211-214, 224, 226,
       230
    pediatric, 356
Ventricular quadrigeminy, 171-172
Ventricular rate, 3° AV block and, 249-250
Ventricular response, 176
    to atrial fibrillation, 105-106, 140
    slow, 7-8
Ventricular rhythm, 201-202
    regular, 252
Ventricular salvos, 167-168
Ventricular standstill, 232
Ventricular tachycardia (VT), 7-8, 167-168, 177-180,
      181-182, 184, 185-186, 202, 226, 230, 336,
      342, 349-354
    axis and, 335-336
    effect of carotid sinus massage on, 138
    escape rhythms vs., 201-202
    history and, 335-336
    morphology of, 335-336
    non-sustained, 177-178, 179-180
    pediatric, 356
    pulseless, 24, 186
    slow, 204

    statistics and, 335-336
    sustained, 177-178, 179-180, 186
    true, 204
Ventricular trigeminy, 171-172, 174, 345-346
Ventriculophasic sinus arrhythmia, 246
Verapamil, 8, 108, 114, 124, 132, 298, 310, 312
VT; *see* Ventricular tachycardia

W

Wave
    fib, 104, 105-106, 112
    P; *see* P wave
    T, 17-18, 70
    U, 17-18
WCT; *see* Wide-complex tachycardia
Wenckebach block, 84, 261-262, 263-274
    footprints of, 265-268, 271-272, 274, 285-286
       pediatric, 366
    pediatric, 365-366
Wenckebach periodicity, 268
Wide-complex tachycardia (WCT), 7-8, 180, 181-182,
      184, 214, 336, 341
      342, 350, 352, 354
Wolff-Parkinson-White (WPW) syndrome, 312

Rapid Locator Guide